THE INNER HEART OF REIKI

I am a Tendai monk, the founder of Tendai Sect, Denkyo Daishi Saicho, which stresses Doshin – Heart for the Way – as of most importance. In *Denjyutsu Isshin Kaimon*, Kojo (Tendai monk, 779–858) quotes Saicho's famous words: "There ⁑ ⸒elihood in Doshin, there is Doshin in livelihood."

I had the opportunity to spend a w⸒ ⸒e upon his visit to Japan, when I had tʰ ⸒ough Buddhist practices. I wa⸒ ⸒ Frans' Doshin and was struck wiᵗ

In high regards to Frans S ⸒ ⸒ave presented him with the Kesa – monk's stole – ⸒ ⸒ceived upon initiation to priesthood. Kesa is the soul of ⸒ priest. Having witnessed his Doshin and soul, both in person and through *The Inner Heart of Reiki: Rediscovering Your True Self*, I look forward to Frans' further endeavors.

Reiki is not merely a "technique," but has a vital role in guiding one to reach "perfection as a human being." The idea contained in the precepts, "Just for today, do not anger, do not worry…" also is reflected in *One Day, One Life* by my teacher, Sakai Yusai Dai Ajari.

If you want to know whether a teacher is a true Reiki teacher or not, all you have to do is to ask him what the True Self is. Without the trustworthy insight of the True Self, nobody can insist he or she is a true disciple of Mikao Usui. This book testifies that the author is one of the true Reiki teachers.

Takeda Hakusai Ajari

The Inner Heart of Reiki resonated deeply within me, for I have always believed that we are all one and that Oneness is the essence of our universe. In this book Frans Stiene takes us on a journey through Japanese Buddhist teachings and meanings of mantras and kanji as taught by Mikao Usui. It is a journey back to our True Self, Oneness and being Reiki rather than living in duality and just doing Reiki. This book is a must-read not just for Reiki Practitioners and Teachers but for everyone who is on life's journey of discovery. So much of Frans' research, study, and practice are openly shared with the reader. Frans does not just talk the talk; he genuinely walks the walk.

The Australian Reiki Connection Inc. is pleased to endorse *The Inner Heart of Reiki* to its members and to the Reiki community.

John Coleman, president of Australian Reiki Connection Inc., Australia's leading Reiki association

Every once in a while you find a book that changes everything. It is almost like you have a paradigm shift, and you take the words into your new understanding of how the world could be. Things that you always questioned come clearer even though you did not know that there was confusion. Frans Stiene's new book *The Inner Heart of Reiki* is just such a book. Every page took me deeper into myself and lit up the places where there were shadows of doubt about the system of Reiki and the spiritual path that I am on.

I have studied Buddhism for a number of years and have been working on becoming a Zen priest for the past few years. I also have a yoga studio and have trained in yoga for the past 20 years. Neither Zen nor yoga have been able to take me as close to my true nature as Reiki has done. When asked what religion I am, I say I am a Reiki Buddhist for that reason.

In Buddhism there is a well-renowned sutra called the Diamond Sutra. It is called the Diamond Sutra because it cuts through delusion. This book is similar in that it cuts through the delusion and hype of typical Reiki books and goes right to the core of what Reiki really is, a spiritual path. This book hits the mark and the mark, it turns out, is the true self.

Frans has gone further than anyone in the world to study and learn about the system of Reiki and it shows on every page, always bringing us back to our True Self, inviting readers to explore for themselves what the true essence is all about. We are fortunate that Frans has done the research for us and we can all follow the path that he has cleared for us.

I have decided that I will not teach anyone the third level of Reiki unless they have read this book, because if they have not we cannot have a good conversation of what the deeper elements of the system of Reiki are, so there would be no reason to advance anyone to that level.

Jeff Emerson, Reiki and yoga teacher, author of *Unfolding the Lotus*

This is a must-read for all students of the system of Reiki. Frans, through his research and practice, has peeled away the myths about the system of Reiki and gives us a clear understanding of the Reiki journey. He also shows how meditation practice is a fundamental part of the system. This book is just what the Reiki world needs, written by someone who walks his talk.

Helen Galpin, co-founder of the British School of Meditation

Having investigated The Great Way of the Asians in shamanism, Daoism, Buddhism, medicine, ancient science, Tai Chi and Qigong since 1963–4, I have a special appreciation of any "system" that articulates the natural presence of the truth and power of the Universe within a context of Self. Versions of self-discovery, self-awareness, ultimate personal potential and the revelation of the True Self – from Lao Zi and Daoists, to Shakyamuni and the Buddhist flourishing, to the great Zen monks and poets – all point to the same views, insights and practices. Mikao Usui's Way is one of those beautiful articulations of the mastery of the nature of human experience and the True Self. Frans Stiene has done us a huge favor by revealing the actual context of Reiki as a Way of Self-Cultivation which is primarily focused on refinement of self which happens to include a method of helping and healing others that is a secondary feature of The Way.

Dr. Roger Jahnke, OMD, founder/director of the Institute of Integral Qigong and Tai Chi (IIQTC); author of *The Healer Within* and *The Healing Promise of Qi* http:/IIQTC.org

Frans Stiene is an inspiring teacher because he embodies the spiritual gift of Reiki in all his actions and throughout his day, not just when giving someone a session. In this delightful book he weaves the threads of the rich history of Japanese spiritual practices that have brought him to this inner sacred space.

Neil McKinney, MD, author of *Naturopathic Oncology*

Frans Stiene is one of the world's premier Reiki teachers and this book is a window into one of his amazing classes. One of Frans' special gifts is to make extremely profound spiritual truths easily accessible. This book will awaken readers to the deeper possibilities of their Reiki practice and offer techniques to help them get there. A must-read for anyone interested in Reiki practice!

Kathleen Prasad, founder of Animal Reiki Source, president of Shelter Animal Reiki Association

The Inner Heart of Reiki is a wonderful companion for the advanced Reiki student and/or teacher who wants to dive deeper into their daily practice and expand their energetic understanding of Reiki. This book is a clear and concise guide to help you integrate the various components of the system of Reiki – the precepts, meditations, symbols/mantras, and hands-on-healing – into your sessions, classes, and most importantly, your life.

Frans Stiene, often referred to as "the Reiki Teacher's Teacher," takes his extensive research and grounded personal understanding and practice, and outlines a path of practice you can follow in his gentle, compassionate, and often humorous way.

As a Reiki teacher and practitioner, I found this book quite breathtaking. Breathtaking is the perfect word – this book reminds you to connect to your breath and your True Self while reading it! The book was truly wonderful, and something I'll reread and refer to often as I expand my personal understanding of Reiki.

Deborah Flanagan, Reiki teacher and author of *Building a Powerful Practice: Strategies for Success to Create Your Wellness Business*

The empathetic way Frans Stiene described the soul of the system of Reiki shows that he is able to understand the true meaning of being yourself.

Ben Midland, author of *The Sacred Mirror*

Frans Stiene illuminates the intricacies of Reiki with the insight and simple elegance of a master. His writing resonates with the depth of experience.

Barry Lancet, award-winning author of *Japantown*

Frans Stiene opened my eyes to the original teachings of the system of Reiki – and allowed me to finally grasp the ultimate depth it offers. I am forever grateful for this. Frans' authentic and inspirational approach allows students to really embrace Reiki – their True Self – in their everyday lives. It is fair to say that his way of teaching brought the understanding of the system of Reiki to a new level in the Western world. His book, *The Inner Heart of Reiki: Rediscovering Your True Self*, is a must-read for all Reiki practitioners and teachers.

Torsten A. Lange, director of the Reiki Academy London and author of *Reiki: Heal Your Body and Your Life with the Power of Universal Energy*

The Inner Heart of Reiki

Rediscovering Your True Self

The Inner Heart of Reiki

Rediscovering Your True Self

Frans Stiene

AYNI
BOOKS

Winchester, UK
Washington, USA

First published by Ayni Books, 2015
Ayni Books is an imprint of John Hunt Publishing Ltd., Laurel House, Station Approach,
Alresford, Hants, SO24 9JH, UK
office1@jhpbooks.net
www.johnhuntpublishing.com
www.ayni-books.com

For distributor details and how to order please visit the 'Ordering' section on our website.

Text copyright: Frans Stiene 2014

ISBN: 978 1 78535 055 9
Library of Congress Control Number: 2015932896

A CIP catalogue record for this book is available from the British Library.

Design: Stuart Davies
Cover calligraphy: "Rising Dragon" by Michiko Imai

Printed and bound by CPI Group (UK) Ltd, Croydon, CR0 4YY, UK

We operate a distinctive and ethical publishing philosophy in all
areas of our business, from our global network of authors to
production and worldwide distribution.

CONTENTS

To all my teachers

Full Moon
Your teachings never forgotten
Resonating deeply inside my heart
Thank you Sensei

My teachers are my family, fellow travelers on the path,
humanity, animals, the earth, the sky, space, in fact
everything...

Digging for the Truth – A Glimmer of Hope

A storm blows through my mind,
I am dragged away to the past, present, and future.
Memories are grabbing hold of me like the cold iron fist of
  winter.
Worry engulfs me as if I am drowning in a lake,
and the fear is overwhelming.
My energy is shaking like a shorn sheep in the bitter night of
  early spring.
Yet deep underneath all of this turmoil in my confused,
  turbulent mind I can see a glimmer.
A glimmer of hope.
I need to dig deep underneath the soil,
getting my hands dirty,
leaves in my hair,
a kind of wild look on my face,
as I dig deeper than I ever have.
But the more I want this glimmer, the deeper I need to dig;
it never seems to stop.
This glimmer of hope keeps eluding me as if I am trying to
  grasp air with my bare hands.
Each time my hands close, I peek inside as if I finally got it,
but nothing is there.
I am tired of digging, tired of the storm in my mind,
tired, oh so tired…
I finally give up, my doubt as big as the tallest mountain.
My doubt that I am not strong enough, like an ox, to dig.
I fall on the moss, moistened by my tears, giving up,
and I let go.
The earth starts to shake,
suddenly the clouds depart and the sun shines in all its glory.
My eyes are closed,

a light deep inside,
heat blazes through me,
devouring all my doubt and my turbulent mind.
Layers upon layers are just falling away like castles made of
   playing cards.
Nothing is left; I am naked.
The truth shines right into my heart.
Just Be, just Be, just Be, it is whispering.

Foreword

What is healing? This is a question that we all ask ourselves from time to time, especially when someone we love or we ourselves face a health challenge. Within the last three years in my battle with breast cancer, it is a question that I found impossible to ignore. As a Reiki practitioner and teacher of more than sixteen years – who lives and breathes meditation and healthy lifestyle choices – it became a question so big, so complex and so frustrating that at certain moments it was unimaginable that I could ever answer it. And yet, within the pages of the book you hold in your hands at this very moment, is a very clear, very straightforward, very real answer.

This book is, in one word, extraordinary.

In a sentence: Put on your seatbelt, because this book will change your life.

This is largely because of the amazing human being who wrote it: Frans Stiene. His body, mind and spirit are infused with light, compassion, wisdom and with joy. His healing presence is so expansive and contagious; those of you who have met him or attended a class know what I mean. Those of you who are about to read his words will soon know as well.

I doubt there is another human being on this planet better able to bring ancient Japanese teachings to the modern world. This is a man who is completely devoted to the teachings of Mikao Usui. In fact, Frans has used Reiki practice to heal himself, as well as many others along the way.

Of course I am totally biased. I have known Frans for more than eight years and from the moment I met him, he changed my life. In the beginning, it was all about how I could apply his teachings to my work with animals. The first time I took his class, so many light bulbs were going on for me: "Oh, that is what that dog was telling me." "Oh, that is what that horse was showing me." With Frans' perspective, I now had words to describe the profound healing experiences I had with animals while sitting in meditative Reiki sessions with them. Because of this I became a much better Animal Reiki teacher.

I am also biased because I know that these teachings helped me to beat cancer. Little did I know that within a few years of studying and taking these practices to heart, Frans' teachings would be my guiding light through facing my own impermanence – and facing it head-on, not because I wanted to, but because cancer forced me to. Honestly, I can't imagine how I could have made it through all my cancer surgeries and treatments without the wise and sure guidance of Frans. Without the spiritual support and positivity he radiated. Without the daily (sometimes hourly) meditation practices I had learned from Frans. Today I am strong again. I am healed. And I am 110 percent convinced that Frans' teachings need to be brought to this world because they are *the* antidote for suffering. I am so honored to be introducing this book to you today!

This book is not about how to avoid all of life's difficulties, but rather it is a guide for how to achieve true and lasting healing and wellness, regardless of the outer situations and challenges you may find yourself in. It is an exploration of Mikao Usui's techniques, not only from an intellectual viewpoint, but also more importantly from an experiential viewpoint. Usui-san wanted to teach us about what healing really was, and he left us many clues to this end, many of which are described in detail throughout the book. But more than all of these particulars, this book is an invitation to let go of preconceived notions about life and separateness and expand your consciousness into unity and Oneness.

Let this book be the spark to ignite the flame of passion back into your spiritual meditation practice. This book will show you the way, very simply, back to your own true nature, your inner heart and your deepest essence. Yes, I think Mikao

Usui would be very proud.

Kathleen Prasad
Founder of Animal Reiki Source, co-founder of The Shelter
Animal Reiki Association
Author of *Reiki for Dogs* and co-author of *The Animal Reiki
Handbook* and *Animal Reiki*
San Rafael, CA
February 2015

Preface

In this book I will not go much into the history of the life of Mikao Usui, as you can find this in some of the other books I have co-authored, like *The Reiki Sourcebook, The Japanese Art of Reiki* and *Your Reiki Treatment*. I will also not explain the specific meditations or hand positions, as that has been discussed over and over in many Reiki books. Rather I will go straight to the inner heart of the system of Reiki: how we can rediscover our True Self.

This book could not have been possible without the help of my teachers, but the most important element is that this book would not have been possible without my own personal practice. Because it is only through our own personal dedicated daily practice that we can start to rediscover the real inner heart of Mikao Usui's teachings. Teachers can only point the way, but we have to walk the path ourselves. If we merely repeat the words of our teachers, we have become like parrots and our own teaching will be empty, without a direct experience. Therefore the teachings within this book come from my own understanding, direct experience, and viewpoint of Mikao Usui's teachings. These insights have come about through my research and training with Japanese Shingon, Tendai, and Shugendo priests. If we want to find the inner heart of the system of Reiki we also need to look at traditional Japanese spiritual practices and see how they relate to Mikao Usui's teachings. I have therefore peppered this book with quotes from famous spiritual teachers and teachings, mainly Japanese, so that you can get a clear picture of what the inner heart of the system of Reiki is all about and how all these real teachers point out the same things.

I could have not written this book alone and I would therefore like to thank Hiromi Hayashi for her help with all the Japanese kanji and translations. I would like to thank Rev. Kûban Jakkôin, Reverend Takeda Hakusai, Rev. Jion Prosser, Rev. Reyn Yorio

Tsuru, and Rev. Jiryo Shoden Doshi for their support and teachings. Without them I would not have been able to write this book. Thank you Bronwen for your support and some editing. Thank you Bella for being who you are.

As the title suggests, this book is not only a journey into the inner heart of the system of Reiki but also a journey into your own True Self. So let's join hands and walk this path together.

Part I

The Inner Heart of the System of Reiki

Chapter 1

Reiki Is True Self

The word "Reiki" has been translated in different ways but the real inner meaning of the word Reiki is True Self. Think about it, the word Reiki literally translates as spiritual energy. But then we have to ask ourselves: What and where is this spiritual energy? Is it outside of us, is it inside us, or is it both? If it is outside of us, then we see that spirituality is very external, never looking within, never looking at the real issues. If we think it is only inside us, then we start to forget about others; we become more selfish. But if after investigation we start to realize that spiritual energy is both inside and outside of ourselves, we start to get a much better picture of what it really embodies.

However, we can go even deeper than experiencing that it is both inside and outside of ourselves: we can start to rediscover that this spiritual energy is neither inside or outside of ourselves; it is all-encompassing. Imagine an empty glass jar; we might think that the space inside the jar is very different than the space outside the jar, but what if we take a hammer and smash the jar to pieces? Can we still say what space was inside or outside the jar? No, because the space inside and outside the jar has mingled and we cannot distinguish them; we could say, they have become of one taste. Another word for this experience of "one taste" is non-duality. This non-dual experience is our True Self, who we really are without the boundaries of the ego. This is spiritual energy. This is Reiki, our True Self.

We can also use the image of a chick in an egg; when the chick breaks the shell, the space inside and outside become the same. However, and this is a very important point, the chick breaks the shell from the inside out. This is the same within our own spiritual rediscovery of our True Self: it needs to come from the inside out. This is why all spiritual teachings are about going inwards.

This One Mind that is within you and me is not inside, outside, or in the middle. And at the same time it is inside, outside, and in the middle. Like the stillness of empty space, it pervades everywhere.
– Xunyun, in Sheng Yen, *Attaining the Way: A Guide to the Practice of Chan Buddhism*

However, there is one difficulty within this teaching, and that is that we cannot show someone their True Self. Why not? This is because the True Self, like the space inside and outside the jar, is very difficult to point out. How can we point out space? We can't hold it, it has no color or smell, and so how can we say to someone, "Look, here it is"? Therefore the masters of old used poetry, symbols, rituals, cryptic words and sounds as signposts to point us towards our True Self. Often we forget that these signposts are just that: signposts, pointing us towards our True Self. We often get distracted by the signposts themselves. We start to say things like, "This signpost is so powerful, we always have to use it!" We hug the signpost, never letting it go, instead of looking at where the signpost is pointing to: our True Self. Within Mikao Usui's teachings we find five signposts:

- The Precepts
- Meditation Techniques
- Symbols and Mantras
- *Reiju*/Initiation/Attunement
- Hands-on Healing

All of these five signposts are pointing towards our True Self. This rediscovering of our True Self in Japan is called *anshin ritsumei* or *satori*. By following these signposts, one day we will be like the jar: we will smash through the barrier of separateness and realize our non-dual nature, our True Self. At this point we have become Reiki and our practice moves from "doing Reiki" to "Being Reiki." This is the inner heart of the system of Reiki: how to embody Being Reiki.

When we truly forget the self, there is no division between inside and outside, no division between yourself and externals. In such a way, we can appreciate life in its fullness.
– Taizan Maezumi, *Appreciate Your Life: The Essence of Zen Practice*

Mikao Usui used a wonderful metaphor for our True Self within his teachings and that is our own innate great bright light (Jp. *Dai Kômyô* – the Shinpiden Reiki Level III mantra). Our True Self is always bright no matter what happens. Imagine a lamp with a lampshade over it; if we place more lampshades over the light it looks like the light is diminishing. If we take all the lampshades off, it looks like the light becomes stronger. But in reality the light itself didn't diminish or become brighter, it stayed the same. This is the same with our True Self, our great bright light. When we practice the meditation practices it looks like our light becomes brighter, and when we get angry, for example, it looks like our light diminishes. But in reality our light is always bright. We might say that during our practice we become clearer, or that we can connect to more energy, but from the viewpoint of our True Self, our great bright light, there is nothing to enhance or improve. To realize this straight away is very difficult. Mikao Usui understood this too, and therefore he created a specific system of teachings so that one day we can lay bare our great bright light.

So the old Gakkai members said that Usui Sensei taught the way to Satori very intensely to those who had achieved a certain level.

– Hiroshi Doi, *A Modern Reiki Method for Healing*

Let's go back to the image of a lamp with many lampshades. What if we start to take the lampshades away – what will happen? It looks like our light becomes brighter, but what else? Our light becomes great, because each time we take a lampshade away our light will shine out farther and farther. This has a huge impact on our compassion to others, because now our light will be able to touch all sentient beings. And all sentient beings, if they want, can benefit from this light.

Now we have come to a very important teaching by Mikao Usui, and that is the question, "What is healing?" In many modern teachings the idea of healing has become mainly focused on physical healing. But what is real healing?

The word healing means to make whole. From a spiritual perspective, to make ourselves whole again we need to remember that we are the universe. Or in other words, we need to rediscover our True Self because it is only in that state of mind that we fully realize that the universe is us and we are the universe. Mikao Usui pointed this out within his precepts. His precepts are all about the mind. He pointed out that if we heal the mind, the body will follow. The deepest level of healing for ourselves is therefore to rediscover our True Self, and the deepest level of healing others is to help them to rediscover their True Self.

Within the precepts we have the precept, "Show compassion to yourself and others." Remembering our True Self is the most compassionate thing we can do for ourselves, and helping others to remember their True Self is the most compassionate thing we can do for them. Rediscovering our True Self is all about letting go of the "I" or the ego, because it is the "I" who is in the way of remembering that we are the universe. This is why the precepts are all about letting go of the "I." Thus the precepts also point out the journey to remember our True Self.

> Everybody worries about the body, its beauty and its health. We worry too much. Diseases are partly the by-product of the ego. So we have to begin by healing our ego. Be open. Abandon the ego, and illnesses can be neutralized in advance. Following the cosmic order is the best preventative therapy for body and mind, the healthiest.
> – Taisen Deshimaru, *Mushotoku Mind: The Heart of the Heart Sutra*

Because Japan borrowed kanji (written characters) from China, it is also interesting to look at how the kanji of "Reiki" is seen from a Chinese traditional viewpoint. The kanji of Reiki in Chinese becomes Ling Chi. My Taoist teacher, Li Ying, told me that from a Taoist perspective Ling Chi is the Tao, or in other words our True Self. She stressed that this kind of energy can only be accessed through serious meditation practice.

> Ling Chi is the subtlest and most highly refined of all the energies in the human system and the product of the most advanced stages of practice, whereby the ordinary energies of the body are transformed into pure spiritual vitality.
> – Daniel Reid, *Chi Gung: Harnessing the Power of the Universe*

Chapter 2

Usui Reiki Ryôhô

The common name used for Mikao Usui's teachings is *Usui Reiki Ryôhô*.

Reiki = True Self
Ryô = to cure or heal
Hô = method or dharma, teachings, truth

Usui Reiki Ryôhô can be read as: Usui's teachings (dharma) to cure and heal one's True Self. Of course Mikao Usui is using a metaphor: to heal one's True Self. He knew that there was nothing to heal – we just need to remember our True Self. However, if we say to people, "Just remember your True Self," they might get confused. Due to all our lampshades we might think that just remembering our True Self is way too easy and wouldn't work. Thus we need to use the word "heal" as a metaphor. To heal is to make whole, thus we can also say: Usui's teachings (dharma) to remember the wholeness of one's True Self. We might be able to remember our True Self for a very short moment in time, but then the lampshades take over again and our great bright light looks as if it has vanished. Thus we need specific practices that help us to remove these lampshades once and for all.

This Dharma (ho, "truth") is amply present in every person, but unless one practices, it is not manifested, unless there is realization it is not attained.
– David Edward Shaner, *The Bodymind Experience in Japanese Buddhism*

The name "Reiki" describes a healing system to rediscover your

True Self and doesn't say anything about hands-on healing. The name itself provides the clue that it is only through the rediscovery of our True Self that we can start to do hands-on healing on others at a much deeper level. Mrs. Takata, who brought the system of Reiki to the West, also pointed out that Reiki starts with rediscovering the "energy" of the True Self. Mrs. Takata's diary, dated 10 December 1935, says that the

> meaning of "Reiki" Energy within oneself, when concentrated and applied to patients, will cure all ailments – it is nature's greatest cure, which requires no drugs. It helps in all respects, human and animal life. In order to concentrate, one must purify one's thoughts in words and meditate to let the true "energy" come out from within. It lies in the bottom of the stomach about 2 inches below the navel. Sit in a comfortable position, close your eyes, concentrate on your thoughts and relax.

Here she is saying that Reiki is the energy within oneself; she even calls it the True Energy, which lies at the bottom of the stomach. She is emphasizing that we need to concentrate and meditate to let the energy come from within. She was pointing out already the heart of the system of Reiki; however, most of these teachings by Mrs. Takata have been lost and are not taught in many of her teachings.

By looking at these clues we can see the importance of the system of Reiki as a method of rediscovering our True Self before we could even think of helping others. The Usui Reiki Ryôhô Gakkai (Society of Usui's Teachings to Cure and Heal One's True Self) in Japan also concurs:

> First we have to heal our spirit. Secondly we have to keep our body healthy. If our spirit is healthy and conformed to the truth, the body will get healthy naturally.
> If you can't heal yourself how can you heal others?

means "peace in your heart/mind," and if we have found pe[ace in] our heart/mind then we can start to help others find this pea[ce in] their heart/mind. This is the ultimate kindness. This is [the] ultimate healing. This is rediscovering our True Self.

> Heart is simply heart. Mind, a key term in Buddhism, is [a] synonym for the same thing.
> – Taizan Maezumi, *Appreciate Your Life: The Essence of Ze[n] Practice*

[T]he following quote from Hiroshi Doi's book, *A Modern Reiki [M]ethod for Healing*, offers us some insight into how the concept of [a]nshin ritsumei fits into Usui's teachings:

> Usui Sensei personally selected, from among qualified Okuden Koki level students, those who possessed a high level of spirituality, and offered them further instructions at Shinpiden level. Shinpiden students were selected to receive Usui Sensei's direct private teachings and learn how to aim for Anshin Ritsumei.

[A]s we can see, Mikao Usui was selecting students for his deeper [te]achings, students who were ready to go to the inner heart of his [te]achings. These were students who understood that healing had [to] start with our heart/mind, because when our mind is clear our [bo]dy and energy become clear as well. These were students who [un]derstood that his teachings were all about rediscovering the [Tru]e Self. We will delve deeper into these deeper elements in [o]ther chapters in this book. We often get so sidetracked with [ph]ysical healing that we start to forget the heart/mind aspect [wh]ich is pointed out by the precepts.

[T]here are many different translations of the precepts; again [one] is not better than the other, just a different way of looking at [them.] We will explore the precepts later in this book; however,

> – "Reiki Ryôhô Hikkei," a manual handed out by the Usui Reiki Ryôhô Gakkai

From these clues we can see that we must start with the self in order to rediscover the True Self, and this is the ultimate healing journey. For me, Usui Reiki Ryôhô is a spiritual practice whose teachings help us to move from not knowing our True Self to knowing our True Self.

> Everything in the Universe possesses Reiki without any exception.
> – Note from a student of Mikao Usui from Hiroshi Doi's manual

When we start to rediscover our True Self we also start to see that everything else is made up of this great bright light: a person, an animal, a rock, a blade of grass, everything. And if everything is a great bright light then we are all interconnected. If we discover this we also have the direct experience of compassion, because pure compassion only takes place when all things are included. Many people claim to be in the direct lineage of Mikao Usui, and that they are teaching the "true" teachings of Mikao Usui. But is this possible? This is an interesting question since it is said that Mikao Usui taught different students different things depending on their spiritual progress.

> Usui Sensei had no standard curriculum, and the length of time of the training depended on the spiritual progress of each student. It is said that he gave one-on-one lectures mainly on the right mental attitude needed for spiritual advancement based on his own experience.
> – Hiroshi Doi, *A Modern Reiki Method for Healing*

This means that different teachers are teaching different aspects of

Mikao Usui's teachings and these will relate to the teacher's own personal understanding, as well as the particular teachings given by their Reiki teacher, their teacher's teacher, and so on. For example, one teacher might focus on a clinical hands-on healing method, and another teacher may emphasize the spiritual aspects of Mikao Usui's teachings. These different "ways" with Reiki indicate each teacher's own personal interest. In addition, Reiki students will gravitate to the teacher who speaks to their own spiritual understanding, progress, and "way." One is not better than the other, just a different path. In addition, each practitioner's unique contemplation, practice and experience of the tools they are given is much deeper than lineage and teacher, as it consists of a simple and direct experience of Mikao Usui's teachings, which is for me his real heritage and lineage. Despite these differences related to each Reiki teacher and practitioner's uniqueness, it is also interesting to think about what Mikao Usui, himself, had in mind.

> ...although the style may still exist, it is difficult to know in many cases what the founder's original intentions were, how he expressed himself to his students, or if the style has indeed changed over the centuries. What prompts or handbooks still exist may mean very little to the uninitiated and sometimes even to the current teacher himself.
> – William Scott Wilson, *The Swordsman's Handbook: Samurai Teachings on the Path of the Sword*

In this book I'd like to take a look at the tools Mikao Usui left behind and see what clues about his teachings we can find hidden within these tools. To understand better Mikao Usui's tools I'd like to attempt to see them from a late 1800s to early 1900s perspective, rather than a modern Japanese outlook. Taking a historical perspective is an important way we can try to see things with his eyes so we can more deeply investigate the clues he left behind.

Chapter 3

The Precepts and Our True Self

The system of Reiki is often called a system of healing, is "healing"? As I've mentioned earlier, to "heal" does only to physically heal ourselves but most important our heart/mind. This kind of healing is about rediscov True Self, the deepest healing of all. Fortunately, Mika us the precepts, central to the system of Reiki, which kind of healing out as well. The following version of th is from the Usui memorial stone, a translation found Doi's manuals:

> Just for today,
> Do not be angry
> Do not worry
> Be thankful
> Do what you are meant to do
> Be kind to others

Within the precepts, whatever version we may be co Mikao Usui is pointing to the heart/mind element t is our True Self. He is not saying anything about a p and we can see that helping others is not mentione precept. First he states that we need to heal ou anger and worry, because these are obstacles th from helping others. And what does helping Healing them on a physical level? If that were the have pointed this out in the precepts as well. No towards helping others to get rid of their anger to find their True Self. In other words the prece out *anshin ritsumei* – spiritual peace, or enligh ultimately the precepts are there to help point out the way to ultimate healing: the path to our True Self. My personal favorite form of the precepts is below. It is said that Mikao Usui taught these to his Buddhist students.

Do not bear anger, for anger is an illusion
Do not be worried, for fear is a distraction
Be true to your way and your being/True Self
Show compassion to yourself and others
Because this is the center of Buddhahood

This form of the precepts takes the healing of our mind even a step further as it discusses illusion, distraction, and Buddhahood. It makes sense that Mikao Usui may have given different students slightly different versions of the precepts to support their spiritual progress and understanding. Also at the time of Mikao Usui, Buddhism was not in favor as everybody had to be State Shinto, especially people in public service, like the navy for example. So it makes perfect sense that Mikao Usui would have taken out the more Buddhist teachings of his system when he started to teach people like Chujiro Hayashi. But no matter what translation we use, in reality they all point out the same: rediscovering our True Self.

The precepts are not only the foundation of the system of Reiki but also the outcome of practicing the system of Reiki. When we have fully embodied or "become" the precepts, we have at the same time rediscovered our True Self. It is in the state of mind of our True Self that we have no more anger and worry, are true to our way and being, and are truly compassionate. This is the center of Buddhahood, the center of Mikao Usui's teachings, and the center of our True Self. In other words, this is the center of real healing.

Chapter 4

Hara/Tanden

The *hara* or *tanden* is a very important element within the inner heart of the system of Reiki. But what is the *hara* or *tanden*? Literally the word *hara* means abdomen; *tanden* means field of elixir or ocean of ki (energy). But as with most Japanese kanji, there are many hidden meanings. The hidden meaning of both *hara* and *tanden* is that they are our true center. Some teachers use the word *hara*, others *tanden*, but when we get caught up in words or debating if it is called this or that, it takes us away from our true center.

> The notion of tanden in Japan (often referred to by the vernacular hara 腹) is of central importance to its performance arts and martial arts, where it is taught that the physical and mental energies should be gathered there, rather than in the head, shoulders, or other points of the body.
> – Charles Muller, *Digital Dictionary of Buddhism*

The *hara* is a concentration point used in most of the practices within the system of Reiki, and it is situated approximately three finger widths below the navel. It's best to visualize the *hara* as closer to the spine than the surface of our belly, as this will bring our concentration point inside of our body. It is through developing our center that we can start to rediscover our True Self. Why do we concentrate on this area of our body? If we stand up and touch our lower belly we see it is the center of our physical body. We can see it is our center of physical balance. In addition, what do we often say when we do not feel well within ourselves, emotionally or physically? We might say, "I am off center, or off balance today."

– "Reiki Ryôhô Hikkei," a manual handed out by the Usui Reiki Ryôhô Gakkai

From these clues we can see that we must start with the self in order to rediscover the True Self, and this is the ultimate healing journey. For me, Usui Reiki Ryôhô is a spiritual practice whose teachings help us to move from not knowing our True Self to knowing our True Self.

Everything in the Universe possesses Reiki without any exception.

– Note from a student of Mikao Usui from Hiroshi Doi's manual

When we start to rediscover our True Self we also start to see that everything else is made up of this great bright light: a person, an animal, a rock, a blade of grass, everything. And if everything is a great bright light then we are all interconnected. If we discover this we also have the direct experience of compassion, because pure compassion only takes place when all things are included. Many people claim to be in the direct lineage of Mikao Usui, and that they are teaching the "true" teachings of Mikao Usui. But is this possible? This is an interesting question since it is said that Mikao Usui taught different students different things depending on their spiritual progress.

Usui Sensei had no standard curriculum, and the length of time of the training depended on the spiritual progress of each student. It is said that he gave one-on-one lectures mainly on the right mental attitude needed for spiritual advancement based on his own experience.

– Hiroshi Doi, *A Modern Reiki Method for Healing*

This means that different teachers are teaching different aspects of

Mikao Usui's teachings and these will relate to the teacher's own personal understanding, as well as the particular teachings given by their Reiki teacher, their teacher's teacher, and so on. For example, one teacher might focus on a clinical hands-on healing method, and another teacher may emphasize the spiritual aspects of Mikao Usui's teachings. These different "ways" with Reiki indicate each teacher's own personal interest. In addition, Reiki students will gravitate to the teacher who speaks to their own spiritual understanding, progress, and "way." One is not better than the other, just a different path. In addition, each practitioner's unique contemplation, practice and experience of the tools they are given is much deeper than lineage and teacher, as it consists of a simple and direct experience of Mikao Usui's teachings, which is for me his real heritage and lineage. Despite these differences related to each Reiki teacher and practitioner's uniqueness, it is also interesting to think about what Mikao Usui, himself, had in mind.

> ...although the style may still exist, it is difficult to know in many cases what the founder's original intentions were, how he expressed himself to his students, or if the style has indeed changed over the centuries. What prompts or handbooks still exist may mean very little to the uninitiated and sometimes even to the current teacher himself.
> – William Scott Wilson, *The Swordsman's Handbook: Samurai Teachings on the Path of the Sword*

In this book I'd like to take a look at the tools Mikao Usui left behind and see what clues about his teachings we can find hidden within these tools. To understand better Mikao Usui's tools I'd like to attempt to see them from a late 1800s to early 1900s perspective, rather than a modern Japanese outlook. Taking a historical perspective is an important way we can try to see things with his eyes so we can more deeply investigate the clues he left behind.

Chapter 3

The Precepts and Our True Self

The system of Reiki is often called a system of healing, but what is "healing"? As I've mentioned earlier, to "heal" doesn't mean only to physically heal ourselves but most importantly to heal our heart/mind. This kind of healing is about rediscovering our True Self, the deepest healing of all. Fortunately, Mikao Usui left us the precepts, central to the system of Reiki, which points this kind of healing out as well. The following version of the precepts is from the Usui memorial stone, a translation found in Hiroshi Doi's manuals:

> Just for today,
> Do not be angry
> Do not worry
> Be thankful
> Do what you are meant to do
> Be kind to others

Within the precepts, whatever version we may be contemplating, Mikao Usui is pointing to the heart/mind element that in essence is our True Self. He is not saying anything about a physical issue, and we can see that helping others is not mentioned until the last precept. First he states that we need to heal ourselves of our anger and worry, because these are obstacles that prevent us from helping others. And what does helping others mean? Healing them on a physical level? If that were the case he would have pointed this out in the precepts as well. No, he is pointing towards helping others to get rid of their anger and worry, and to find their True Self. In other words the precepts are pointing out *anshin ritsumei* – spiritual peace, or enlightenment. *Anshin* means "peace in your heart/mind," and if we have found peace in our heart/mind then we can start to help others find this peace in their heart/mind. This is the ultimate kindness. This is the ultimate healing. This is rediscovering our True Self.

> Heart is simply heart. Mind, a key term in Buddhism, is a synonym for the same thing.
> – Taizan Maezumi, *Appreciate Your Life: The Essence of Zen Practice*

The following quote from Hiroshi Doi's book, *A Modern Reiki Method for Healing*, offers us some insight into how the concept of *anshin ritsumei* fits into Usui's teachings:

> Usui Sensei personally selected, from among qualified Okuden Koki level students, those who possessed a high level of spirituality, and offered them further instructions at Shinpiden level. Shinpiden students were selected to receive Usui Sensei's direct private teachings and learn how to aim for Anshin Ritsumei.

As we can see, Mikao Usui was selecting students for his deeper teachings, students who were ready to go to the inner heart of his teachings. These were students who understood that healing had to start with our heart/mind, because when our mind is clear our body and energy become clear as well. These were students who understood that his teachings were all about rediscovering the True Self. We will delve deeper into these deeper elements in further chapters in this book. We often get so sidetracked with physical healing that we start to forget the heart/mind aspect which is pointed out by the precepts.

There are many different translations of the precepts; again one is not better than the other, just a different way of looking at it. We will explore the precepts later in this book; however, ultimately the precepts are there to help point out the way to ultimate healing: the path to our True Self. My personal favorite form of the precepts is below. It is said that Mikao Usui taught these to his Buddhist students.

Do not bear anger, for anger is an illusion
Do not be worried, for fear is a distraction
Be true to your way and your being/True Self
Show compassion to yourself and others
Because this is the center of Buddhahood

This form of the precepts takes the healing of our mind even a step further as it discusses illusion, distraction, and Buddhahood. It makes sense that Mikao Usui may have given different students slightly different versions of the precepts to support their spiritual progress and understanding. Also at the time of Mikao Usui, Buddhism was not in favor as everybody had to be State Shinto, especially people in public service, like the navy for example. So it makes perfect sense that Mikao Usui would have taken out the more Buddhist teachings of his system when he started to teach people like Chujiro Hayashi. But no matter what translation we use, in reality they all point out the same: rediscovering our True Self.

The precepts are not only the foundation of the system of Reiki but also the outcome of practicing the system of Reiki. When we have fully embodied or "become" the precepts, we have at the same time rediscovered our True Self. It is in the state of mind of our True Self that we have no more anger and worry, are true to our way and being, and are truly compassionate. This is the center of Buddhahood, the center of Mikao Usui's teachings, and the center of our True Self. In other words, this is the center of real healing.

Chapter 4

Hara/Tanden

The *hara* or *tanden* is a very important element within the inner heart of the system of Reiki. But what is the *hara* or *tanden*? Literally the word *hara* means abdomen; *tanden* means field of elixir or ocean of ki (energy). But as with most Japanese kanji, there are many hidden meanings. The hidden meaning of both *hara* and *tanden* is that they are our true center. Some teachers use the word *hara*, others *tanden*, but when we get caught up in words or debating if it is called this or that, it takes us away from our true center.

> The notion of tanden in Japan (often referred to by the vernacular hara 腹) is of central importance to its performance arts and martial arts, where it is taught that the physical and mental energies should be gathered there, rather than in the head, shoulders, or other points of the body.
> – Charles Muller, *Digital Dictionary of Buddhism*

The *hara* is a concentration point used in most of the practices within the system of Reiki, and it is situated approximately three finger widths below the navel. It's best to visualize the *hara* as closer to the spine than the surface of our belly, as this will bring our concentration point inside of our body. It is through developing our center that we can start to rediscover our True Self. Why do we concentrate on this area of our body? If we stand up and touch our lower belly we see it is the center of our physical body. We can see it is our center of physical balance. In addition, what do we often say when we do not feel well within ourselves, emotionally or physically? We might say, "I am off center, or off balance today."

We must therefore keep our mind firmly at the center of our body that is the center of our true self, to avoid its falling into a state of imbalance.

– Motohisa Yamakage, *The Essence of Shinto: Japan's Spiritual Heart*

Bringing our mind and therefore our energy back to this center helps us to become stable and balanced. If we focus on the *hara* more and more, this will create a stability that becomes a solid foundation for the rest of the teachings to build upon. Imagine a big tree with hardly any roots, yet this tree has grown a big canopy. What happens if some external wind comes along? The tree falls over. The same can be said for a mountain: the mountain has a solid base and not a narrow, pointy one. Nothing ever grows from the heavens downwards; everything grows from the earth upwards to the heavens. We are also a part of nature; we need to grow upwards from the earth with a solid foundation and not the other way around. Another image is an upside-down pyramid. An upside-down pyramid is very unstable and this is a metaphor for what can happen energetically if we focus solely on developing our head or third-eye area; we become off center.

We put our mental concentration in the hara. The hara is a point in our body that generates chi, energy, and it is approximately two inches below the navel.

– Taizan Maezumi, *Appreciate Your Life: The Essence of Zen Practice*

To nurture this foundation Mikao Usui taught *joshin kokyu hō* to his beginner students. During *joshin kokyu hō* we focus on the *hara* so that we start to become more centered and stable. When we are centered and stable we start to remember our connection with the earth and our physical body. Once Usui's students had a solid foundation, they were allowed to take Okuden Level II, in which the foundation was solidified by working with the first symbol and the mantra, *choku rei*. We will look at this mantra later in the book but for now it is sufficient to say that these tools stimulate the *hara* and therefore take our foundational work even further.

Aikido, another Japanese spiritual system, also sees the *hara* as the foundational practice:

Ueshiba-sensei stated, The foundation of aikido is within becoming empty like the sky. From this standpoint, the freedom of harmonious movement is born. Becoming empty means to discard all illusory thinking and mistaken ideas of self. The highest consciousness (gokui) of aikido is to blend one's movement with the invisible world of spirit, the kototama. This being accomplished the entire universe is contained in your hara, the vital center from which new life energy is born.
– William Gleason, *The Spiritual Foundations of Aikido*

Mrs. Takata pointed out the importance of this center as well in her own teachings. She wrote, "In order to concentrate, one must purify one's thoughts in words and meditate to let the true 'energy' come out from within. It lies in the bottom of the stomach about 2 inches below the navel." Mrs. Takata taught that our true energy comes out of this center. We can also see this in Buddhist teachings:

[*hara*], located just below the navel, is the true center of the person, and the proper seat of the mind. True mind.
– Charles Muller, *Digital Dictionary of Buddhism*

We can see the importance of the *hara* as well within the precepts:

Do not bear anger, for anger is illusion.
Do not worry, for fear is distraction.
Be true to your way and your being.
Be compassionate to yourself and others,
for this is the center of Buddhahood.

What happens when we get angry? What is happening with our energy? The energy of anger shatters our stable foundation and moves the energy upwards and in all directions. To gain control of this angry energy we need to make sure it can't explode in all directions. This is done by bringing our awareness into the *hara*, which stabilizes our destructive energy. The upward energy of anger might cause headaches, high blood pressure, stress, excessive talking, redness on the skin, etc. However, this doesn't mean that we should bottle it up. It means we simply need to focus on our *hara* when we are angry, for by focusing on our *hara* we are becoming mindful and no longer follow our anger. The anger may come up, but it will dissipate all by itself because when we focus on the *hara*, the anger has no one feeding it. In other words when our mind turns away from the anger, it starts to dissolve back into our true center, our True Self.

What about worry? We worry because we are not in the present moment. Perhaps we are anxious about something in the past or worried about a future possibility. Thus we have lost our center and our energy is scattered. We must again bring our minds to our *hara* when we feel worried. In this way we stop feeding the worry so that it can dissolve on its own. Focusing our worried minds on the center of our being, our *hara*, helps bring it back into balance.

How does this relate to the third precept? Can we be true to our way and our being (our True Self) if we are worried, angry and fearful? No, of course not! When we are being true to our way and being, we are not carried away by emotions and our energy can stay balanced.

Energetic balance will show itself in our lives by the compassion we have for ourselves and others. Compassion flows easily from a centered and balanced person. Compassion is the purpose of our True Self.

The last precept mentions the center of Buddhahood. In order to embody Buddhahood, or our great bright light, we need to be solid and centered in our body. Our body is the vehicle in which we rediscover our great bright light. So it is through the *hara* that we can embody our True Self. In other words, to become the great bright light – Dai Kômyô – we need to go through the *hara*, our true center.

There is another hint to the *hara/tanden* within one version of the precepts which says, "心身 改善 *Shinshin kaizen* – Improve your heart/mind and body." Yuasa Yasuo, in his book *The Body, Self-Cultivaion, and Ki-Energy*, states that the word *shin* 心 also has the same meaning as *tanden*: "ocean of ki." So Mikao Usui was pointing out the importance of the *tanden* if we want to improve our heart/mind and body.

The kanji of *shin* 心 is also found with the third mantra, *hon sha ze sho nen*. One of the meanings of this mantra is "I am Right Mind." Thus Usui is showing us that to reach a state of Right Mind we need to go through the *tanden/hara*.

Mind and *hara* are often used together in Japanese daily language in phrases like:

hara wo sueru – to make up one's mind

or

hara de kangaeru – to think with one's *hara*

If we go deep into the heart of the system of Reiki we will start to rediscover three energy centers within our own being:

下丹田 *ka tanden* – below *tanden/hara* (below navel)
中丹田 *chu tanden* – middle *tanden* (middle of chest/heart)
上丹田 *sho tanden* – upper *tanden* (forehead)

First we need to develop the *hara*, just below the navel, as this is the foundation for the other two centers. This is why the *hara* is in fact the most important one; without a well-developed *hara*, it will be very difficult to develop the other two centers. Mikao Usui knew this too and that is why he taught practices which focus on the *hara* in Shoden. He found it so important that even the first symbol and mantra he taught in Okuden Level II focused on the *hara* before the others were introduced. The upper *tanden* is traditionally connected to *sei heki*, the second mantra taught within Okuden Level II. The middle *tanden* is traditionally connected to *hon sha ze sho nen*, the third mantra taught in Okuden Level II. And when these two centers start to merge completely with the center of the lower *tanden*, we start to remember our True Self, great bright light, Dai Kômyô or soul:

> The spiritual content of aikido can be expressed in the one word hara, which ranges in meaning from "belly" to "heart-mind" or "soul." Hara is not only the physical center of the body; properly understood, it is also the center of our spiritual energy.
> – William Gleason, *The Spiritual Foundations of Aikido*

We can also explore the specific sounds inside the mantras as taught within the system of Reiki to find more hints to these three energy centers, and a deeper experience of *hara*. There are so many hidden meanings to be found within Mikao Usui's teachings, and this is also why practicing the system of Reiki is a lifelong journey. We can only really discover these elements within ourselves if we gain a direct experience by practicing all the meditation techniques.

Chapter 5

Mind, Body, Energy

One of the important elements within Mikao Usui's teachings, and for that matter in many Japanese spiritual teachings, is the concept of mind, body, and energy/speech. In Japanese these are called *sanmitsu*, which translates as the three mystic practices.

Mind = *i mitsu* = mental mystic practice – mandala
Body = *shin-mitsu* = bodily mystic practice – mudra
Energy/Speech = *ku mitsu* = verbal mystic practice – mantra

They are called mystic as they are very difficult to understand. They are mysteries, like Shinpiden, the mystery teachings. Only a direct experience can unravel the mystery. Shinpiden is the mystery of the universe so within this we see *sanmitsu*; one cannot exist without the other. Ultimately we need to merge with the mind, body, and energy of the universe, or in other words we need to realize that our mind, body, and energy is the same as the universe mind, body, and energy. This unification is realizing our union with the great bright light, Dai Kômyô, which in essence is connected to a deity called Dainichi Nyorai. This connection to the deity will be discussed later. However, from a traditional Japanese spiritual perspective, when we unify with the three mysteries we unify with Dainichi Nyorai. Thus within the heart of the system of Reiki we can start to see many interesting connections which will guide us to rediscover our True Self.

If a practitioner is able to cultivate the proper actions in accord with the three mysteries and join in communion with the Nyorai, then he has attained enlightenment in this very body.
– David Edward Shaner, *The Bodymind Experience in Japanese*

28

Buddhism

We could say that in our normal everyday life our mind, body, and energy have become conditioned. This conditioning comes from our upbringing, society, influences, you name it. Each person will be conditioned differently depending on many factors, which in turn create labeling and judgment. This is why we cannot say "This is hot" or "This is cold" – it completely depends on the condition of the person saying this.

Mitsu also means intimacy, just like the kanji of kindness in the precepts. We will discuss intimacy in more detail later in the book. The intimacy of *sanmitsu* is about working towards being intimate with our own mind, body, and energy as it is only then that we can become one, or intimate, with the mind, body, and energy of the universe.

> It is further conceived ontologically that all sentient beings possess by nature the same mystic forms of action as the Buddha's – as it is technically called "無相の三密" (*muso no sanmitsu*) – but they do not realize them until they successfully perform the prescribed method of practice and attain unity with the Buddha.
> – Kukai, *Shingon Texts*

If we look at the system of Reiki we can see these three mysteries clearly represented.

The mind contains visualizations which are the symbols, but the mind is also the intellectual element of the precepts. Body is represented by the hand positions for ourselves and others, but also the position we sit in to do the meditation practices, and the movements we do during the *reiju*/initiation/attunement. Energy is always linked to speech, which in turn are the mantras within the teachings, but also the chanting of the precepts. As you can see, Mikao Usui clearly based his teachings around the philosophy of mind, body, and energy.

Let's go into the inner heart of *sanmitsu* in relation to the system of Reiki.

Mind

Mind is the most important element within these teachings. Mikao Usui also pointed this out in the precepts. The precepts are not about the body or energy, but all about the mind. Mind rules our body and energy. If our mind is not clear, our body and energy is also not clear. Here are a few very simple examples to help us see that the mind rules our body and energy. A dead person has a body yet cannot move – why? Because the person's pure mind, True Self, has left the body. Thus we can see that if there is no mind, the body does nothing. This is the same with energy or speech. A dead person still has a mouth but can't speak. Mind is often the hardest to understand as it is the most subtle of the three. We can feel our body, it is not that difficult; we can connect to or feel our energy, but the mind is very subtle. The mind doesn't have a specific location, shape, sound, etc. This is also why Mikao Usui added body and energy practices to his foundational mind teachings of the precepts. He realized that for many of his students this was very difficult to embody, hence the meditation practices he created that focused on the body and energy.

Master of secret, how to attain wisdom?
Know one's mind as it truly is.
– Dainichi-kyo Sutra

As the mind is the most important, we need to understand that within hands-on healing we need to have the right mind. Without the state of right mind our energy goes all over the place. This means our body will get quickly tired as well. Our mind affects our body and energy. Think about how an angry person walks.

His anger is first of all in his mind, but what kind of effect does it have on the body? And another example: If you get a client who is insecure, worried and fearful, how does she lie on the table? Her insecurity, worry and fear is in her mind, but when she lies on the table her body is tense. How about a person who is angry: does he speak nicely or not? By investigating this we can start to see how the mind influences our body and energy. The ultimate meditation is resting our mind in the great bright light of our True Self. But that is very hard for most beginners, thus we use visual aids like symbols. In the end we need to let go of the symbols, otherwise they will become obstacles.

Away with all images. The great meditation of void is to be our companion.
– Kukai, *Shingon Texts*

Body

Body is very important as it is the vessel for finding our True Self; we need to embody spirituality. If the vessel is not solid or the right way up then we cannot pour anything into it. This is why in Mikao Usui's teachings we focus on the *hara* and on the quality of earth energy. This is all about creating a solid base, a stable vessel for embodiment of our True Self. The word "embodiment" points already towards the body. This means we have to accept our body, become intimate with it, because if we discard it we can never find this embodiment.

Without forsaking his body, one attains supernatural power over the real world, wanders freely on the ground of great space, and perfects the mystery of Body.
– Dainichi-kyo (Mahavairocana Sutra)

As the body is the most physical of the three it is easier to practice with for many people. This is why hands-on healing has become so popular. Many people find it much simpler to perform hands-on healing than to contemplate the mind practices like the precepts, for example. The mind is very elusive, it has no form, shape, or color, but the body does and thus it is much easier to work with.

Energy or Speech

Energy is also speech; for speech to develop we first need to have a thought, this thought triggers the inner energy through our channels, and this energy makes a vibration in the channels that creates sound. This is why speech is connected to the breath, so speech is also seen as the in-breath, the out-breath and the pause in between. Energy is seen as the link between the mind and the body, going from gross to subtle to even subtler. This also means that within the progression of your practice within the system of Reiki, you move from more bodily practices to energy/speech practices to finally mind practices.

So you begin this study by training the ch'i by means of technique. After your beginning studies, you will discipline your ch'i, but move away from technique.
– Issai Chonzanshi, *The Demon's Sermon on the Martial Arts*, translated by William Scott Wilson

The energy or speech practices within Mikao Usui's teachings are mantras to be chanted over and over again while you sit in a meditation posture. Mantras are tools to become mindful; they help us to not get distracted by the past, present, and future.

Meditate upon it [the sound] until you become united with it. Then you will attain perfection.
– Kukai, *Shingon Texts*

Within Japanese esoteric teachings the main sound is often the sound of A. This sound is connected to a deity called Dainichi Nyorai which in turn is connected to the mantra Dai Kômyô, as taught by Mikao Usui. When we embody the cosmos we embody Dainichi Nyorai, as Dainichi Nyorai is the personification of the cosmos.

In Our Practice

If our mind is tense it will be hard to visualize things; if our body is tense it is hard to perform hand positions; if our speech is tense we cannot sound mantras. If our mind is too loose it is the same, therefore we need to be right in the middle, not too loose or too tense. We also have to realize that mind, body, and speech are not separate from each other but intertwined. All these three mysteries are interrelated to each other and need to be in harmony. In the end we need to realize that everything is mind – a mandala, everything is body – a mudra, and everything is energy/speech – a mantra. When we start to realize this, we will be getting closer to the inner heart of the system of Reiki and our lampshades start to fall away, exposing our True Self.

The mantras as taught by Mikao Usui are also interlinked with the three mysteries. *Choku rei* is connected to the body aspect, *sei heki* is connected to the energy/speech aspect, *hon sha ze sho nen* is connected to the mind aspect, and finally Dai Kômyô is connected to the embodiment of the three mysteries as a whole. For example, a direct translation of *hon sha ze sho nen* is, "I am Right Mind." This is pointing towards the mind aspect of the three mysteries. Ever wondered why the first two symbols are clearly symbols and the second two are in reality kanji? That is because the first two are tools to help us to remember our pure earth and heavenly energy within us. And the latter two are both indicating a state of mind.

When the mind, body, and speech become more and more subtle, our practice will become subtler as well. We all know that if our mind is tense our hand positions will become tense. So if our mind becomes less tense and more open, our hand positions become more open and expanded as well. We might even move away from physically touching the person. In fact if the client and the teacher are both having a clear mind, body, and energy they can just sit opposite each other and remember their state of mind of interconnectedness. Imagine a frozen lake, which represents our disconnectedness from our mind, body, and speech. If we throw a pebble on the frozen lake there will be no ripple effect. Now imagine a lake that is not frozen and very calm; this represents being in harmony with our mind, body, and speech. Throw a pebble in this lake and you will get a huge ripple effect. The more we gain a direct experience of the three mysteries, the calmer our mind becomes and the greater the ripple effect will be. What does that mean? It means that we can set the intent of hands-on healing or *reiju*/initiation/attunement and it is already happening without the need for the body or energy/speech practices to become involved.

We can also observe how our students are connecting to their mind, body, and energy. While performing a hands-on healing session, how is the stance – is it sloppy? If so, that means that the mind and energy are also sloppy. Is the stance stable? If so, that means that the mind and energy are also stable. How is our student sitting during a meditation practice or how is she performing a *reiju*/initiation/attunement? By observing this as a teacher we can help our students to go deeper into the heart of the system of Reiki as we can guide them better.

If we are interested in taking our practice into the heart of the system of Reiki, we need to be aware of how this will affect our own mind, body, and energy. Sometimes our mind takes a huge leap and our energy and body needs to catch up. Sometimes our energy takes a huge leap and our mind and body needs to catch up. And sometimes our body takes a huge leap and our mind and energy needs to catch up. Here are a few examples: You start to chant the mantra and suddenly you get some physical symptoms.

This indicates that your body is not completely ready so it needs to catch up with the energy flow that is being triggered by the chanting of the mantra. Or after many months practicing the mantra, we suddenly might find that we want a little break from it and we focus more on reading spiritual books. We might have had an energetic experience and now our mind needs to catch up with reading about it and how it relates to us. We can also experience this in hands-on healing on others. Some practitioners might find that when they do hands-on healing they get a pain in their arms or hands; often this is blamed on the client's negative stuff or healing, but in fact it is you. The pain is inside of you, not inside the client, so what is it? It is your meridians that are expanding during a hands-on healing session; they are not used to a sudden influx of energy coming through them and they expand; this in turn triggers a bodily/physical sensation such as pain in the arm or hand. This experience is pointing out that our body is not ready. If that happens, we need to prepare our body better through practice so that it can embody the fullness of the energy.

Mind, body, and energy also point to different practices. Let's look at one of the precepts; for example, "Do not be angry." The practice for the body would be to renounce our anger; we try not to be angry at all, and we see it as something bad. However, the practice for energy is to transform the anger into something else, the desire to do a meditation practice for example. We can do this because we realize that the underlying energy of anger or not being angry is the same and thus we can transform that energy into something else. If we do not have a direct realization of this underlying principle then it becomes hard to do. The mind practice is the hardest of all because the mind practice is based on non-duality, our True Self, the heart of the system of Reiki. Our pure mind is like a mirror – it reflects everything – but it doesn't label what it reflects as good or bad, thus we do not get angry. This kind of mind practice is cutting the root of anger; it is the heart of Mikao Usui's teachings. However, this is not as easy as it sounds and this is why within the system of Reiki there are mind, body, and energy practices. Depending on the student's spiritual progress, he or she would use more mind, body, or energy practices. We can clearly see this within a *reiju*/initiation/attunement; if both the teacher and the student are at the level of mind then there is no need for bodily movements, visualizations, or energy practices, but only mind-to-mind connections.

Chapter 6

Meditate to Rediscover Our True Self

In order to be the best Reiki practitioner and/or teacher we can be, we must dedicate ourselves to a daily practice. What might this practice be? According to Hiroshi Doi, the meditations of *joshin kokyu hō* and *hatsurei hō* are some of the most important elements within Mikao Usui's teachings.

We humans hold the Great Reiki that fills the Great Universe. The higher we raise the vibration of our own being, the stronger the Reiki we have inside will be.
– Note from a student of Mikao Usui from Hiroshi Doi's manual

This quote helps to explain why Mikao Usui put meditation practices like *joshin kokyu hō* and *hatsurei hō* within the system of Reiki. The more we practice them, the stronger our Reiki will become. In fact, *hatsurei hō* literally means, "generating a greater amount of spiritual energy." Therefore we can see that Mikao Usui was pointing out that regular practice of this meditation would generate a greater amount of spiritual energy. In turn we can use this energy for helping ourselves and others to redis-cover the True Self. By simply trying these meditations once, we do not get anywhere; we need to practice these meditations on a daily basis. Through regular practice with these meditations, Mikao Usui was pointing us again back to the precepts. As a result of our dedicated meditation practice, we will begin to let go of our anger and worry and become more compassionate to ourselves and others.

A dedicated meditation practice also means that we need to repeat again and again the same practice because it is only out of repetition that we start to embody the specific meditation practice. We need to do it again and again and again. This is in fact the same with everything we do. If we only practice playing the guitar once, we get nowhere, but if we play it once a day we start to grow and one day we "become" the instrument. Repetition also helps us to learn from our mistakes; each time we do it, we can slowly and subtly adjust the practice until we do it perfectly. We all know the saying "practice makes perfect," but that is not the right saying! We can practice the practice in an incorrect way and thus it doesn't become perfect. This saying is in fact "perfect practice makes perfect." One of the side effects of repetition is to help make our practice perfect.

Nowadays people do not like to repeat things. They claim too quickly that they get it. Sure, maybe superficially, but then they forget just as quickly.
– Taisen Deshimaru, *Mushotoku Mind: The Heart of the Heart Sutra*

The more we repeat the practices, the deeper we go; the deeper we go, the more organic the practice will become. If we learn to play the guitar and we still play it like when we started 10 years ago then that means we haven't grown, we haven't become organic. This is the same with anything else we do in the world. The teachings need to become organic. Dedicated practice will help you to become more natural and organic to your own True Self. We can see this too within the precepts:

Do what you are meant to do.
[or]
Be true to your way and your being.

Being true to our way and our being/True Self means to become organic. We can copy the teacher but if we do not make it our own then we are copycats of the teacher, and we become true to his way and not our way. Our practice needs to become our own: an expression of our True Self, fluid and organic.

It means when you become you, yourself, and when you see things as they are, and when you become at one with your surroundings, in its true sense, there is true self.

– From a lecture by Shunryu Suzuki

Part II

The Precepts

Within the system of Reiki we use a set of precepts. The precepts are the foundation of the system of Reiki and they are also seen as instructions. They instruct us how to practice hands-on healing, how to use the mantras and symbols, how to do the breathing practices, and how to use the *reiju*/attunement/initiation.

Many different translations of the precepts exist; one is not better than the other, just a different translation. Why the differences? Kanji can be translated in many different ways and it also depends on the spiritual understanding of the person doing the translation. By going deeper into the translation, we can discover the inner heart of the precepts.

> A Shingon master, Master Kobo, said that one kanji contained a thousand meanings.
> – Taisen Deshimaru, *Mushotoku Mind: The Heart of the Heart Sutra*

Often only the surface meaning (*omote* in Japanese) of the system of Reiki is taught; however, the International House of Reiki always tries as much as possible to teach the inner/hidden meaning (*ura* in Japanese) of the teachings of the system of Reiki. When we teach the *ura* of Mikao Usui's teachings we will gain a much deeper understanding and therefore also a more direct experience of his teachings. Let's look at the *ura* of the Reiki precepts.

Ultimately the precepts are not just words to recite; we need to embody the precepts in all that we do. Then they become even more dynamic and free-flowing, and in this way we can start to see how the precepts relate to our own direct experience and in fact every aspect of our lives.

When we maintain the precepts and the spirit of the precepts in how we walk, how we sit, how we eat, how we talk, and how we relate to one another and to our environment, their constant presence brings light to our lives.

– Jakusho Kwong, *No Beginning, No End: The Intimate Heart of Zen*

Chapter 7

Translation of the Precepts from Usui's Handwriting

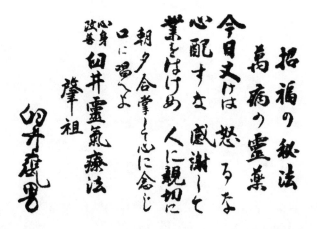

It is said these precepts are written by Mikao Usui. However, there is no full proof of this. I personally also believe that since Mikao Usui was teaching his students according to each person's spiritual progress, he would have also given them precepts to match each person's different understanding.

招	福	の	祕	法
shou	*fuku*	*no*	*hi*	*hou*
invite	blessings	of	secret	method

萬	病	の	靈	藥
man	*byoo*	*no*	*rei*	*yaku*
10,000	illnesses	of	spiritual	medicine

今日	丈けは	怒る な		
kyo	*dakewa*	*ikaru na*		
today	only	anger not		

心配	すな	感謝	して
shinpai	*suna*	*kansha*	*shite*
worry	not	gratitude	do

業 を はけめ	人	に	親切	に
gyo o hageme	*hito*	*ni*	*shinsetsu*	*ni*
practice diligently	people	to	kindness	be

朝夕	合掌	して
asayuu	*gassho*	*shite*
morning and evening	gassho	perform

心	に	念じ
kokoro	*ni*	*nenji*
heart/mind	to	pray silently

(deeply bearing in the heart/mind)

口	に	唱へ よ
kuchi	*ni*	*tonae yo*
mouth	at	chant do

心身	改善
shinshin	*kaizen*
heart/mind and body	reform/improve

臼井靈氣療法
Usui Reiki Ryôhô

肇祖	臼井甕男
Choso	*Usui Mikao*
Founder	Usui Mikao

Chapter 8

Exploring Some of the Kanji

Blessing: *Fuku*

Fuku 福 is often translated as blessing, and many people see this blessing as an external element. It is a blessing that someone does for you, like the *reiju*/initiation/attunement. However, in reality it is a blessing we connect with within ourselves. This blessing happens when we start to embody the precepts, when we let go of our anger and worry, and when we start to become more grateful and are showing more compassion to ourselves and others. This blessing is the inner spiritual rain that will start to happen when we go deeper into our True Self.

From a Buddhist perspective *fuku* also means the rewards we encounter from practicing the dharma. What are these rewards? These rewards are many but we can boil it down to one, and that is rediscovering our True Self. In Buddhism this reward is called merit, thus the basic meaning of *fuku* is merit. This merit is often interlinked with the six paramitas, which we will discuss in a later chapter. Was Mikao Usui already saying that by embodying his precepts we are also starting to embody the six paramitas?

Secret Method: *Hihō*

In the first line of the precepts, we can see the kanji 祕法 *hi hou* or *hihō*, translated as secret method or secret rituals. Breaking down the translation further, we can see 祕 *hi* which means secret, hidden, esoteric, spiritual, deeper, and 法 *hō*, which means dharma, reality, true principle, original nature, original essence. The following quote from one of my Japanese teachers sheds even more light on the inner *ura* meaning of *hihō*:

The expression hihô is used often by Buddhist people to

45

speak about "the most important teachings." Around 1900 is the end of the Meiji period, which was against Buddhism precepts in Japan. I think Usui Sensei wanted his students to remember that to follow the six paramitas was the most important at this time. The paramitas are the "keys" to develop "bodaishin" which is the Way to be One with Universal Energy. Always think about the hard periods (Meiji, Taisho) in which Usui Sensei wrote and taught. It is very important to reflect like anthropologists do.

– Reverend Kûban Jakkôin, Shugendo priest

The use of *hihō* indicates that Mikao Usui was emphasizing that the precepts are the most important teachings within his system. For me, this shows us that the whole system of Reiki is based on embodying the precepts within oneself and one's life, not just about hands-on healing for others; the true aim of the system of Reiki is rediscovering our True Self or enlightenment. Compassion for others grows from the precepts because it is only when we start to find our own inner True Self that we can really start to help others.

Hihō also points to specific practices within the system of Reiki that nurture awakening to the True Self. In the *Dictionary of Japanese Buddhist Terms* by Hisao Inagaki, *hihō* is described as an "esoteric method of practice, the same as shubo." In turn, this book explains that *shubo* "refers to an esoteric ritual in which a practitioner makes an offering to a deity, recites spells, makes a manual sign and meditates on the deity as prescribed."

Perhaps *hihō* is referring to certain secret rituals in esoteric Buddhism that are based on Sanmitsu. Sanmitsu means, "The Three Mysteries of Mind, Body, and Speech," and refers to one's spiritual development. As discussed previously, we can see these three elements within Mikao Usui's teachings. Practices that cultivate the mind are the visualization of the symbols, specific visualizations during the breathing techniques, and contemplating the precepts. Practices that cultivate the body are the hand positions on yourself or others, sitting in meditation in a specific position, and the ritual of *reiju*/initiation/attunement. And of course the practices that cultivate speech are the chanting of the mantras and the precepts.

Perhaps Mikao Usui used 祕法 *hihō* to indicate and honor his own personal training within esoteric Buddhism. And maybe Mikao Usui created the system of Reiki based on his own personal Japanese esoteric Buddhist teachings and made them more accessible for others. *Hihō* also links to Shugendo practices, such as Mikao Usui's mountain experience.

All of these retreats in the mountains occur for a set length of time during which various ascetic practices are cultivated, culminating in the transmission of secret lore (hiho 秘法) or performance of initiations.
– Miyake Hitoshi, *Religious Rituals in Shugendo*

We can see a link to the Shugendo practice of Fudo in the system of Reiki as well. Within Shinpiden we learn the Dai Kômyô, which is linked to the Buddhist deity Dainichi Nyorai, who is the cosmic Buddha. Dainichi Nyorai is often depicted as Fudo Myoo when he appears on earth to help people rediscover their True Self or reach enlightenment. When Dainichi Nyorai moves on earth he does so in the form of Fudo Myoo. We will discuss these kinds of teachings in a later chapter.

In addition to fire ceremonies, Shugendo rituals include many ceremonies (shuho 修法) utilizing mudras (in 印) and spells (shingon 真言; dharani) for the purpose of realizing the attainment of one's prayers. These ceremonies address certain deities; buddhas such as Yakushi 薬師 and Amida 阿弥陀, bodhisattvas such as Monju 文殊 and Kokuzo 虚空蔵, various forms of Kannon 観音, various Myoo such as Fudo, Indian deities such as Benzai-ten 弁財天, Japanese kami such as kojin, Inari, and Daikoku. An examination of the ceremonies listed in Shugendo manuals show that these ceremonies are most often addressed to the Myoo or the Indian deities and their retinue, with Fudo Myoo the most common figure.

– Miyake Hitoshi, *Religious Rituals in Shugendo*

In conclusion, we can see that the mention of *hihō* in the first line of the precepts shows us that Mikao Usui was pointing to many hidden *ura* meanings in even his most simple teachings.

10,000 Things: *Man*

The kanji 萬 *man* translates as "ten thousand, myriad things, everything." 10,000 illnesses implies all illnesses of body, heart, and mind. The phrase "ten thousand things" is often used within Buddhism and Taoism.

The nameless is the beginning of heaven and earth.
The named is the mother of ten thousand things.
– Lao Tzu

Tao gives birth to One
One gives birth to Two
Two give birth to Three
Three give birth to ten thousand things.
– Lao Tzu

By looking at these quotes we can see that "ten thousand things" occur when we are not remembering the Tao, our True Self. When we start to name things, or in other words when we label things, we step away from the Tao, our True Self. So for me Mikao Usui put this kanji in his precepts to tell us that we cannot remember our True Self due to labeling, naming, and not being in a state of oneness, and that this is really the biggest illness of all. Thus the spiritual medicine is to let the blessings of embodying the precepts rain down on us when we refrain from labeling, thus living in a state of As It Is.

Illness: *Byoo*

The kanji 病 *byoo* translates as illness, disease, grief, and distress.

In East Asian, and especially Chan discourse, [病] often refers to a condition of practice gone errant based on mistaken attachment to certain narrow aspects of the teachings.
– Charles Muller, *Digital Dictionary of Buddhism*

Charles Muller is making an interesting statement about 病 *byoo*, illness. He is saying that illness is not really understanding Buddha's teachings, or in other words not understanding the teachings of our ultimate non-dual reality. Thus our real illness is not a physical illness at all, but rather a confused state of mind. This is of course also the reason why Mikao Usui doesn't mention any physical issues in his precepts; his precepts are all about the mind! Thus we can see that Mikao Usui's hidden *ura* teachings about healing indicate that real healing takes place in our minds.

Anger: *Ikaru*

The kanji 怒 *ikaru* translates as anger, being offended, rage. 怒 *Ikaru* can be broken down to 奴 "on top" and 心 "on the bottom." The kanji 奴 (pronounced yatsu) originally was formed to mean "of low stature," referring to slaves and servants. The kanji 心 (pronounced kokoro) means "heart/mind." Thus we could say that anger comes from an underdeveloped heart/mind. We can see that the precepts keep pointing out our heart/mind again and again, as they are the heart of the system of Reiki.

We need wisdom. This wisdom is a function of the human

heart and mind. It is our innate capacity to see beyond the dualistic world of greed and anger, to where we may learn to live in peace and harmony with all beings. This is not to escape the dualistic world. It is to take care of the dualistic world. To do this, you must first calm your mind.

– Dainin Katagiri, *You Have to Say Something: Manifesting Zen Insight*

Worry: *Shinpai*

The kanji 心配 *shinpai* translates as worry. Worry is made up of two separate kanji, 心 *kokoro/shin*, which means heart/mind, and 配 *pai/hai*, which means to arrange or distribute. So we could say that when we worry, our heart/mind energy is not distributed properly. Or we might say that when our heart/mind is scattered and all over the place, this is when we get worried and have no peace of heart/mind. This also indicates that not to worry is a matter of balancing our heart/mind and being focused and mindful.

Whatever you feel, don't worry about it.

– Dainin Katagiri, *Each Moment Is the Universe: Zen and the Way of Being Time*

Grateful: *Kansha*

The kanji 感謝 *kansha* translates as being grateful or to appreciate. It is made up of two kanji, 感 *kan*, which means impression, influence, sensation, emotion or feeling, and 謝 *sha*, which means thank, apologize, refuse, remove, dispel. We could say that real appreciation is when we refuse to be emotional. This in Buddhism is called seeing things As It Is. When we see life As It Is we do not label or judge. Being grateful is about accepting things as they are. We must resist the urge to label things, such as labeling our experiences as good or bad, hot or cold, positive or negative, for when we do so, we are not looking deeply enough into the precepts. For example, sometimes we become attached to the sensations and feelings we experience during a hands-on healing session and/or our meditation practices. If we really want to be grateful during our practice we need to dispel all sensations and feeling and just Be. True gratitude can arise only when we are not attached to our feelings and emotions.

The kanji 謝 sha can also be broken up so the left side is 言 (to say / words) and the middle and right is 射 (to shoot; that is, an arrow with the implication of piercing, rather than shooting someone with a gun). In other words we have to pierce our words with wisdom and compassion. We must pierce them by not judging and labeling, but rather by being honest and humble and by letting go of anger and worry. This kind of piercing can only come from our True Self, because it is within the True Self that we find our innate wisdom and compassion. Within the imagery of shooting the arrow we see another element as well. As soon as the arrow is shot, all the tension in our body and in the bow is released; thus by being grateful about what we have and who we are, by accepting things as they are, we release all our pent-up emotions and relax. In doing so, we will become less angry and worried.

The kanji 謝 sha also means to apologize. When we apologize there will be a sense of gratitude within the other person. In Japan people often say sumimasen, "I am sorry," in lieu of "thank you" and gratitude.

We express our gratitude toward ourselves as well as toward everything, not as two separate things but both as one life.
– Taizan Maezumi, *Appreciate Your Life: The Essence of Zen Practice*

Practice: *Gyo*

The kanji 業 *gyo* translates as action, karma, business, vocation, arts, strive, endeavor, performance, training, work, practice, skill. *Gyo* is a very important element in many Japanese spiritual practices.

> "Who am I?" "What is a human?" "What is life?" These are questions we forget to think about when we live a life filled with contentment and happiness. I am convinced that if we want to answer these questions, we need to rouse to action and take the challenge of embarking on a gyō.
> – Ryōjun Shionuma, *The Life-long Spiritual Journey of an Apprentice Japanese Bonze: Awakening to a New Worldview by Fulfilling the One-thousand Days Trekking Practice on Mt. Ōmine*

業 *Gyo* has often been translated as work, but for me this is not in line with the rest of the precepts. Work is often seen as something we do from 9 to 5, and by using the word "work" we suggest that for the rest of the day it doesn't matter if we are angry or worried. For many people work is also separate from other things, like being with friends or going to a movie. By using the word work, we are putting the precepts into a box, and not integrating them into everything we do. Practice is something we can do all the time, especially as it relates to letting go of anger and worry.

> For mountain ascetics, gyō is to live according to the spirit of that precept.
> – Ryōjun Shionuma, *The Life-long Spiritual Journey of an Apprentice Japanese Bonze: Awakening to a New Worldview by Fulfilling the One-thousand Days Trekking Practice on Mt. Ōmine*

The kanji 業 *gyo* can also translate as an art form. From a traditional Japanese perspective, an art form is only mastered after hard and long training, like that of a sword maker, a Zen Master, or a Sushi chef. Mikao Usui used this kanji to show us that to really embody his teachings we need to keep training and persevere, and this is a lifelong journey. A *reiju*/initiation/

attunement is not enough; we must also sit down and do our meditation practices so that we embody the precepts to the fullest.

I can say the same about my understanding of life. For me life is not about "me" living and doing something. For me life and gyō are fundamentally an experience of thanksgiving. As I experience it, life is simply a gift I am grateful for. I have never felt that gyō or life was a selfish search for discovering in myself hidden virtues and then exhibiting them like one exhibits trophies.

– Ryōjun Shionuma, *The Life-long Spiritual Journey of an Apprentice Japanese Bonze: Awakening to a New Worldview by Fulfilling the One-thousand Days Trekking Practice on Mt. Ōmine*

Kindness: *Shinsetsu*

The kanji 親切 *shinsetsu* is translated as kindness. *Shinsetsu* is made up of two kanji: 親 *shin* which means intimacy, friend, family, self, in person, affection, parent(s), affection or to experience personally, and 切 *tsetsu*, which means to cut, deep, profound or intimacy. This kindness is about others and yourself. What is interesting to note is that both kanji of kindness also mean intimacy, so we have double intimacy. Say a knife comes in contact with a certain object to be cut. At this moment the knife and the object are both intimate with each other, no separation; who is touching whom? Therefore real kindness is when we become intimate with ourselves and others.

Being one is the activity of intimacy.
– Taizan Maezumi, *Appreciate Your Life: The Essence of Zen Practice*

This kind of kindness can only be real when we cut out the "I," which means that the essence of this kindness is compassion.

When we act kindly from our "I" ego we have many strings attached; we do it because we want something in return. Mikao Usui's teachings are all about rediscovering your True Self, so we need to let go of these strings; we need to cut them, hence the second kanji.

So in essence this precept can be translated as: "Be kind to yourself and others." If we look at it from a spiritual point of view, in conjunction with Mikao Usui's teachings, we can also say: "Be compassionate to yourself and others." If we think it is only to others we are mistaken, and if we think it is only to ourselves we are also mistaken. One's True Self includes everything else, and everything else includes our True Self; this is the heart of the system of Reiki. Intimacy is One with everything.

Dogen Zenji defines doing good as to realize your true self.
– Taizan Maezumi, *Appreciate Your Life: The Essence of Zen Practice*

The kanji 親 *shin* also means parent(s), and thus we can ask ourselves: What do parents do? We can find this by looking at the foundation of this kanji: 立 (*tatsu* – to stand) on top of the 木 (*ki* – tree) to 見 (*miru* – see/observe/be on the lookout) for their child. This of course we can again only do when we feel intimate within our family.

To take care of other beings is to take care of your life in its totality.
– Dainin Katagiri, *You Have to Say Something: Manifesting Zen Insight*

Non-duality: *Gassho*

合掌 *Gassho* literally means putting your palms together, but the deeper meaning is non-duality, the unification of the two opposites. Mikao Usui was pointing out non-duality already within his precepts. Thus, morning and evening one should perform *gassho*, to remember one's non-dualistic nature.

Heart/mind: *Kokoro Ni Nenji*

Kokoro ni nenji 心に念じ translates literally as "heart/mind to pray silently." In essence it means deeply bearing the precepts in your heart/mind. This means to become the precepts, to embody them in your heart. Again Mikao Usui is pointing to our heart/mind within the precepts, the symbols and mantras, the meditation practices, the *reiju*/initiation/attunement, and even within hands-on healing. We should embody the precepts in our hearts/minds because, when we do so, we have rediscovered our True Self, which will affect all the other meditation practices we will perform.

When you observe the precepts without trying to observe the precepts, that is true observation of the precepts.
– Shunryu Suzuki, *Not Always So*

Pray Silently

念じ translates as pray silently. This kanji also means to have in mind or to be mindful about. In other words, be mindful about the precepts in our heart/mind.

Shinshin Kaizen

心身 *shinshin* translates as heart/mind and body. 改善 *kaizen* translates as improve and rectify.

Mikao Usui is saying that we have to improve both our heart/mind and our body. But the deeper meaning of it is that we have to be in harmony with our heart/mind and body, the physical and the spiritual. To become harmonious we need to come from our center; if we are not centered we cannot embody the harmony of heart/mind and body. Thus the first step towards remembering this state is to connect to our other center, the *hara*.

Shin literally means "mind." It also has another implication, which is "center."

– Taizan Maezumi, *Appreciate Your Life: The Essence of Zen Practice*

Usui Reiki Ryôhô

臼井靈氣療法 *Usui Reiki Ryôhô* is often translated as Usui Spiritual Energy Method, but if we look closely at the kanji it can also mean Usui's teachings (dharma) to cure and heal one's True Self.

臼井 – *Usui*
靈氣 – *Reiki* – True Self
療 – *Ryo* – cure, heal
法 – *Ho* – dharma, teachings, method

In Buddhism the Sanskrit term Dharma has three meanings: the ultimate principle of existence, the phenomena of experience, and the teaching about the nature of things. These three meanings work together. For example, without phenomena – without mundane human life – the ultimate principle can never manifest. And unless it is transmitted, the Truth will not be realized.

– Dainin Katagiri, *You Have to Say Something: Manifesting Zen Insight*

By calling his teachings Usui Reiki Ryôhô, Mikao Usui pointed out that his dharma/teachings were about realizing the ultimate principle of existence, realizing our True Self. We need to embody the precepts by sitting down and practicing the meditation techniques as taught within the system of Reiki.

Japanese Insights

According to my Shugendo teacher Rev. Kûban Jakkôin, the teachings pointed to in the precepts are the foundation of the path to self-discovery for Japanese Buddhist practitioners. The precepts point towards virtues we must develop on the path of practicing the system of Reiki. At the time of Mikao Usui, Buddhism was banned, thus Mikao Usui, who was a Buddhist himself, created these simple precepts to help his students to remember to follow the six paramitas. The six paramitas are: generosity, morality, patience, persistence, concentration, and wisdom.

One of my Japanese students sheds more light on the precepts by sharing some insights from Japanese culture:

Shinsetsu and *kansha* are two of the most important virtues of Japanese culture. They are the understated compassion that holds the society interconnected. The understated quality is the key factor. I feel it is the reflective point of humility and humbleness which in turn provokes the search for their place in the society (to be of any benefit to the society no matter how small and to know their humble place in the society) for which being true to what is expected (by the universe) must be contemplated and thus requires one to search for their inner being. So *kansha* is not just a thank-you and *shinsetsu* is not a mere act of kindness.

– Hiromi Hayashi

Hiromi also pointed out to me that the tone of the precepts is that of a grandfather teaching his grandson, full of wisdom and compassion, strict and firm yet nurturing. This again points to an intimate relationship. Mikao Usui was guiding his students this way, so as teachers of the system of Reiki we need to use this kind of teaching style as an example for our own students.

Another of my Japanese teachers offers this insight on the Reiki precepts:

I would summarize the Reiki precepts as reform one's self,

chant, contemplate, show respect, be kind, have gratitude and request blessings. As general categories, these are all common to Buddhism, especially in Japan.

– Reverend Keisho, Tendai priest

In addition, please consider these comments and translation of the Reiki precepts offered by one of my Japanese teachers, Reverend Jiryo Shoden Doshi, a Tendai priest:

The manner in which the "precepts" are written is almost like a Zen koan or quatrain which suggests the whole acts like an introspective meditation. What is this pointing to? It seems one has to kind of "unpick" the order in order to clearly see the meaning. For example:

Practice diligently to be kind.

Morning and evening perform gassho and pray silently.

Chant to reform (cleanse) one's heart/mind and body.

Do not express anger or worry, but give gratitude.

Only when body and mind are purified will the secret method to cure all ills manifest.

Reiki, as I understand it, is not about what one does. "Doing" has very little to do with it. It is more about letting go of the wish or desire for the I to "Do" anything, but rather allow IT to flow. In short, what the Reiki Precepts seem to be saying, in whichever way we read them, is:

One must first correct and surrender Self so that the vessel is purified (Jirki = one's own effort; Gyo practice). Only then will the universal healing spirit flow in (Tariki = other power). The Japanese tend to be more "in tune" with natural environments which surround them in that they see themselves as an integral part of it rather than separate from it as Westerners do. Westerners may tend to say "I am healing." Whereas the Japanese, if they said anything at all, might say "IT heals / Buddha heals / Kami heals," and so forth. The healing process involves the vessel simply as that: vessel.

My Own Translation of the Precepts

In contemplating the inner hidden teachings as well as the Japanese perspectives shared with me, I have created two more translations of the precepts:

The esoteric teachings to invite blessings
The spiritual medicine of having strayed from universal truth:

Today only
Do not anger
Do not worry
Be grateful
Practice this diligently
Be kind to yourself and others

Perform Gassho in the morning and evening
Be mindful about this in your heart/mind
Chant with your mouth
Improve your heart/mind and body

Usui's teachings (dharma) to cure and heal one's True Self
The founder Usui Mikao

And:

The esoteric teaching to invite blessings
The spiritual medicine of having strayed from universal truth:

Today only
Develop your heart/mind (release anger)
Put your heart/mind in order (release worry)
Let go of your attachments to feelings and emotions (be

grateful)
Practice this diligently
Show compassion to yourself and others

Perform Gassho in the morning and evening
Embody this in your heart/mind
Chant with your mouth
Improve your heart/mind and body

Usui's teachings (dharma) to cure and heal one's True Self
The founder Usui Mikao

I hope that these translations provide yet another layer of contemplative thought for those interested in deepening their practice.

When the medicine of Esoteric teachings have cleared away the dust, the True Words open the treasury.
When the secret treasures are suddenly displayed,
All virtues are apparent.
– Kukai, in David Edward Shaner, *The Bodymind Experience in Japanese Buddhism*

Chapter 9

The Precepts on Mikao Usui's Memorial Stone

一ニ	日ク	今日	怒ル	勿レ
ichi ni	*iwaku*	*kyou*	*ikaru*	*nakare*
Firstly	it says	today	anger	do not

二ニ	日ク	憂フル		勿レ
ni ni	*iwaku*	*ureuru*		*nakare*
		(written: *urefuru*, but read as *ureuru*)		
Secondly	it says	sorrow/worry		do not

三ニ	日ク	感謝	セヨ
san ni	*iwaku*	*kansha*	*seyo*
Thirdly	it says	thankful	do

四ニ	日ク	業ヲ	励メ
shi ni	*iwaku*	*gyo o*	*hageme*
Fourthly	it says	practice	diligently

五ニ	日ク	人ニ	親切	ナレ
go ni	*iwaku*	*hito ni*	*shinsetsu*	*nare*
Fifthly	it says	to people	kindness	be

When we compare the memorial stone precepts with the precepts believed to be in Mikao Usui's handwriting, we see two interesting points. The first one is that on the memorial stone the kanji reads *urefuru* – sorrow and not 心配 *shinpai* – worry. This might be due to Mikao Usui giving some of his students a slightly different version of the precepts, all depending on whom he was teaching.

The second thing we can see is that the precepts on the memorial stone are in Kanji and Katakana (different Japanese writing systems) while the handwritten copy is in Kanji and Hiragana. Hiragana gives a much softer impression than Katakana, since Hiragana, originally developed in the 900s, was for personal use, for example *waka* (poetry) and letter writing, not for formal documents. I wonder why this is so? Did Mikao Usui see his precepts as *waka* – poetry? Traditionally *waka* is also seen as 陀羅尼 *darani*, like a mantra.

Kukai (774–835) stated that within *darani* each syllable is a manifestation of your True Self, and that each syllable is symbolic on multiple levels. Therefore once again we can see that connecting to the precepts will help us to rediscover our True Self.

No matter how we translate the precepts, in the end the most important element is to embody the qualities within the precepts. I think that is what Mikao Usui really wanted, so that the people who practice his teachings would gain spiritual freedom.

When we take up the Buddha's Way, the precepts are not seen as rules but as ways to manifest ourselves as buddhas. In our daily life, we must return to the precepts again and again. This effort is very important. It's the effort of simply walking forward, step-by-step.

– Dainin Katagiri, *You Have to Say Something: Manifesting Zen Insight*

Part III

The Reiki Symbols and Mantras

Chapter 10

Choku Rei – True Self

Within Okuden Reiki Level II we use a mantra called Choku Rei 直霊. Let's explore how this mantra is pointing towards our True Self.

Pronunciation

Because Japanese kanji (characters) are derived from the Chinese language, there are two ways to pronounce a kanji. *Onyomi* is the pronunciation that is closer to the Chinese form, typically used for nouns. *Kunyomi* is the traditional Japanese pronunciation, most frequently used when kanji appear in adjectives or verbs. Choku Rei 直霊 is the onyomi pronunciation, while the kunyomi pronunciation of these characters is Naohi (sometimes written as Naobi).While Choku Rei is more commonly known, both are correct; they are just different ways of pronouncing the same kanji. There is only one Japanese Reiki school which uses the pronunciation Naohi and this comes from Mrs. Yamaguchi; she used it in her *reiju*/initiation/attunement. All other Japanese Reiki lineages use the onyomi pronunciation, Choku Rei.

The Meaning of the Mantra

Choku Rei/Naohi/Naobi 直霊 means literally straight, direct, or correct spirit. Some modern Reiki teachers teach that the meaning of Choku Rei is to put the energy straight or directly here or there; in other words when our hands touch a person during hands-on healing, we might focus on the mantra to "put" the energy where our hands touch, making it stronger or more focused in that particular place on the body. This is a very external interpretation and does not reflect the inner spiritual teaching.

From a traditional Japanese perspective, direct or correct spirit describes our True Self; in other words, it describes a way of being where we are able to access our spirit, our True Self, directly. Although in modern Reiki practice Choku Rei might be seen as something we "give" to a person or place, traditionally this was not so; it was an inner, spiritual practice. We can see this more traditional viewpoint about Choku Rei 直霊 in Shintoism and also in traditional Aikido teachings.

Within Shinto being straight/direct is also a very important element as it points towards honesty. We can also see this within the Reiki precept "Be honest" or "Be true to your way and your being." In fact, all the tools within the system of Reiki are just signposts pointing us in the direction of being straight/direct so that we can rediscover our True Self.

The Inner Teachings of Choku Rei

William Gleason is an international Aikido teacher who trained and lived in Japan for many years, and he illuminates a more traditional way of looking at Choku Rei/Naohi/Naobi:

> The central function of naobi is self-reflection: as an intuitive practice, aikido requires constant awareness and assessment of our feelings and intentions. Naobi is the source of both body and mind. It creates the five senses of sight, hearing, smell, taste, and touch and, therefore, individual existence. As life begins with breath, the ki of naobi manifests in the lungs and the skin.
> – William Gleason, *The Spiritual Foundations of Aikido*

We can see in the above quote that traditionally the practice of Choku Rei was done to illuminate one's True Self and was not an external practice. Thus, it is a wonderful practice to use the mantra for remembering our True Self.

We cannot connect others to their True Self; they can only do that themselves. If we could really do this we would have a very different world. This is why using the mantra on others is a very modern interpretation. However, when we remember our own True Self we start to shine our bright light out into the world; in this way we are like a mirror helping others to see their own True Self. This is why Mikao Usui put Choku Rei in his teachings: to help us to remember our own True Self, because this is when real change and real healing can begin.

> When Naobi, the direct spirit, comes into activity, various high-frequency light wave vibrations are emanated.
> – Masahisa Goi, in William Gleason, *The Spiritual Foundations of Aikido*

When I was in Japan in 2012 my teacher, Takeda Ajari, explained that he did the worship of 直日霊 Naohi in the formal service of Shinto during the morning ritual. He would stand and recite mantras in front of a simple wooden shrine that also had a small mirror on it. In one way we might interpret this externally and think this practice is about worshiping at a shrine and focusing on something outside oneself. However, if we look more deeply we can see that the mirror reflects the person who is performing the ritual; so in reality he was performing the ritual for himself, to cultivate a direct/straight spirit so that he might rediscover his own True Self. He explained to me that in Shinto teachings, Naohi is our True Self, our direct correct spirit. By looking in the mirror we also become intimate with ourselves and the more intimate we become with ourselves, the more intimate we will be with the universe.

Seeing Things As They Are

The introspection of naobi is not an abstract process of reflecting on the past. It is to stand in the present and see

things exactly as they are. Naobi is the virtue of makoto – sincerity and gratitude for the gift of life.
– William Gleason, *The Spiritual Foundations of Aikido*

The above quote points to gratitude which we also can find back within the precepts. Here we can start to see a link in how the mantras are interconnected with the precepts. Because practicing with Choku Rei/Naohi/Naobi 直霊 cultivates our True Self, this means that when we work with this tool within the system of Reiki it will help us to see things as they are. What does this mean? Seeing things as they are is about transcending duality; it's about not labeling things that may come up as a result of a hands-on healing session or meditation practice as good or bad, positive or negative, etc. It's about letting go of the idea of a "giver" and "receiver." Seeing things as they are is about seeing from your True Self to the True Self of the other person, animal, tree, or object; the more we cultivate this direct/straight spirit, the more we can connect to all things in life, heart to heart, without any labeling whatsoever. In this way we realize that we are all One.

In your big mind, everything has the same value...In your practice you should accept everything as it is, giving to each thing the same respect given to a Buddha.
– Shunryu Suzuki, *Zen Mind, Beginner's Mind*

Quality

Within the more inner teachings of Mikao Usui this mantra also has the quality of focus. In this case our focus is about rediscovering our True Self without wavering from it. This therefore also becomes a tool for being mindful. When we are talking about being mindful we have to ask ourselves: What do we need to be mindful of? We need to be mindful of not straying from what we are focusing on, in this case rediscovering our True Self. When we stray from what we are focusing on, our mind goes into the three times of past, present, and future. Many modern spiritual teachings talk about being in the now or the present moment. But have you ever tried to pinpoint the now or this present moment? We can't because as soon as we try to pinpoint the now we have already strayed into the past. Therefore real mindfulness is not about the now; rather it is about letting go of the three times, the past, present, and future. The now and present moment is a distraction, because it is in the now or present moment that you think about the past and the future. When we are completely focused we let go of the three times altogether. Focus is therefore also a necessary tool to reach a state of mind of meditation; it is a kind of stepping stone. Before we can walk or talk in a state of mind of meditation, we first need to learn how to stay focused. All the mantras are stepping stones; if we miss one stepping stone we fall into the water and are swept away by all our attachments.

The past is gone, the present is dying, and the future is not yet.
– Sheng Yen, *Attaining the Way: A Guide to the Practice of Chan Buddhism*

The more focused we become, the more we connect to our own innate groundedness; thus this mantra is also about earth energy. If we have no connection to the earth energy within us, we are off with the fairies and therefore we will not be focused but all over the place. Imagine a balloon with a string attached to it. If there is lots of wind, external circumstances, then the wind will take the balloon here, there, and everywhere. The wind represents our fears, distractions and worries which take us away from being focused. But if we tie a stone onto the string of the balloon, the balloon can still move yet it stays where we put it. It is now grounded, connected to the earth; this is like tying the mind to the *hara*, our first step in remembering our True Self.

As we can see, there are many different layers within each mantra, but to really discover each layer we need to chant the mantra again and again and again. Why not just a few times? If you think that the system of Reiki is a spiritual practice that helps you to rediscover your True Self, why stop chanting if you haven't recovered your True Self yet? If you travel from San Francisco and your destination is New York would you stop halfway and stay somewhere? Of course not, you would go all the way. This is the same with the mantras. Go all the way; chant it until you have rediscovered your True Self, for only then can you stop.

Conclusion

As we can see, Mikao Usui, the founder of the system of Reiki, borrowed Japanese spiritual teachings to be placed in his spiritual teachings. When we remember Choku Rei/Naohi 直霊 inner heart, rediscovering our True Self, then we will gain so much more out of our practice. The clearer we know where the tool is pointing, the easier it will be to move in that direction. When we chant these mantras, we take deep breaths so that the sound starts to resonate through our whole being. This kind of deep breathing also stimulates the *hara*, again linking it in with the foundation of the earth energy.

Since we chant these words with energy from the abdomen, it naturally creates the repetition of deep breathing from the belly: this way of breathing is called the "long breathing method" (okinagaho) in Shinto. Through this breathing, the power in the physical body is increased.
– Motohisa Yamakage, *The Essence of Shinto: Japan's Spiritual Heart*

Chapter 11

Sei Heki – True Self

The second mantra used within Okuden Level II is Sei Heiki 性癖 and as with the previous mantra this mantra also points towards our True Self.

The Meaning of the Mantra

In modern practice this mantra has been interlinked with emotional and mental healing. This emotional and mental healing is often seen as letting go of habits we have created such as smoking, drinking, having a specific issue with someone, etc.

But is there a deeper meaning to Sei Heiki? What is the real emotional and mental healing Mikao Usui was pointing out? Before I set out to answer these questions let's take a look at the kanji of Sei Heiki.

Sei 性 means nature, sex, the inner essence of something, innate, inherent, the quality by which one realizes one's True Self, suchness, reality, gender.

Heiki 癖 means habit, manner, kink, vice, trait, indigestion, problem with your spleen, idiosyncracy, inclination.

By looking at the kanji of Sei Heiki we can already start to see a much deeper meaning than just emotional and mental healing.

The Inner Teachings of Sei Heiki

This Self has no shape or form, has no birth, has no death. It is not a Self that can be seen with the aid of your present physical eye. Only the (hu)man who has received enlightenment is able to see this. The (hu)man who does see this is said to have seen into her own nature and became a Buddha. It is to use neither thought nor reasoning and to look straight ahead.

– Takuan Soho, *The Unfettered Mind: Writings of the Zen Master to the Sword Master*

If we look at the translation of the mantra Sei Heiki, we can say that it means: "our inclination to remember our innate True Self." Like the previous mantra, Sei Heiki is pointing to rediscover our True Self. In essence we all want to be happy, we all have an innate drive to be happy; however, we often do not know how to proceed to rediscover this innate happiness. We do not know where to look. We often look to outside ourselves to find happiness: like food, drinking, friends, a good job, Buddha, you name it. However, as Mikao Usui points out, real happiness lies within our True Self. Sei Heiki is yet again another signpost pointing inwards because it is only by going inwards that we start to rediscover our non-dual nature, our True Self.

So let's go back to the question, "What is the real emotional and mental healing Mikao Usui was pointing out with Sei Heiki?" What starts to really change when we are slowly redis-covering our True Self? The answer to this question lies within the non-dual nature of our True Self. Within non-duality we start to soften the grip of our ego, labeling things as good and bad, positive and negative. Inherently things are not good or bad, they are just As It Is. We can only label something as good because we compare it to something bad, and we label something bad because we compare it to something good. So what will happen if we slowly stop comparing things? Our grip on the ego starts to soften; we slowly soften the grip on labeling things as good and bad and start to see them for what they really are. Labeling things as good or bad creates attachments and aversions which in turn creates more and more emotional and mental habits.

Let's look at one of the precepts; for example, "Show compassion to yourself and others." Most of the time we can only be compassionate to the people we like because we label them as good. Yet we will find it very hard to be compassionate to people we do not like because we label them as bad. Thus if the grip on this kind of labeling starts to soften, we become more compassionate, not only to our friends but also to people whom we do not like.

Here is another example: You have to catch a plane and at the airport you hear that the plane has been delayed. If you see this as bad, you will create a lot of anger or worry, but if you see it just as it is, neither good nor bad, then the anger and worry will not transpire. By letting go of these mental habits of labeling things as good and bad we are creating a happier life, not just for ourselves but also for others. This is the real emotional and mental habit we have to let go of, our dualistic labeling. Mikao Usui wasn't pointing out our basic ideas of mental and emotional habits; no, he was pointing to the core, to the heart, the root cause of all our emotional and mental issues: our confused dualistic mind.

Here is another interesting viewpoint about Sei Heki. The word Heiki is also used to indicate that we have an issue with our spleen. In traditional Japanese spiritual teachings, the spleen is associated with earth energy. Our emotional and mental issues all come from over-thinking and analyzing. This means it is associated with the head and heavenly energy, or not being grounded. This in turn means that when our earth energy is not stable, it will have an effect on the spleen. In other words, our energy is being pulled away from our grounding of earth, into the heavenly realm, and therefore depleting the energy of the spleen.

As we saw above, Sei also means sex, which is another interesting element. Traditionally sexual energy is seen as a source for deepening our spiritual practice. This doesn't mean to have sex all the time; it means to use that sexual energy for rediscovering our True Self. We all know, when we feel the need for sex or when we have an orgasm, how much energy is being stimulated. So instead of having sex or orgasms, we can use this sexual energy to fuel our spiritual development. When we have sex, we also feel very intimate and sometimes experience inner bliss; these experiences are all connected to our True Self.

In the view of Eastern meditation, sexual energy is the source of energy for a journey into knowing the ultimate, original human nature.
– Yuasa Yasuo, *The Body, Self-Cultivation, and Ki-Energy*

Quality

In other words, in the realm of pain and suffering, we have to find the realm of peace and harmony. This is religious practice. You cannot find any peace by escaping from human pain and suffering; you have to find peace and harmony right in the midst of human pain. That is the purpose of spiritual life.
– Dainin Katagiri, *Each Moment Is the Universe: Zen and the Way of Being Time*

Within the traditional teachings of Mikao Usui the quality of Sei Heki is harmony.

Harmony has many layers but first of all we need to start to feel harmonious within ourselves, and this we can do by practicing the meditation techniques taught within the system of Reiki. By going inwards, we start to harmonize our own internal energy. In fact, the word Okuden – Inner Teachings – points towards this. We can only harmonize ourselves with the outer elements if we have first harmonized ourselves within. We have to realize that we are the same inside and outside; then we can start to merge with the universe, no separation at all.

Once you have done this and made your mind sincere, the dirt and grime of your ego is naturally brushed off, transforming into a mind that is as pure and undefined as that of a child, removed from all intrusive thoughts. This sincere, uncorrupted mindset, by which you do not worry about anything, is the kind of mind that can reach out to the Buddha and achieve harmony with all things.

– Ryuuzui Nakai, *Ajikan no jisshuu* [Ajikan Meditation Practice]

This kind of harmony is the harmony between the two opposites, good and bad, short and long, hot and cold, you name it. When we rediscover our True Self we will be in harmony with all things. We start to realize that everything we do, every thought we have, has an effect on something. Like the wind that has an effect on the trees: the trees drop their leaves due to the wind blowing through them. Leaves fall on the ground, which will have an effect on the grass and the insects. The leaves on the grass will trigger the right circumstances for mushrooms to grow; now we will pick the mushrooms and eat them. We often think that the wind is just the wind, but in reality the wind triggers lots of things to happen; however, we can only start to see the bigger picture of this if we are in harmony with the wind and all the other elements. This is the same within our own mind; the more we are in harmony, the more we can start to see what kind of effect our mind has on everything else.

Just as Choku Rei is connected to earth energy, so Sei Heki is connected to heavenly energy. Again we can only discover this by using this mantra again and again. If we only use it occasionally when we do hands-on healing on others or on ourselves, we will never discover these hidden meanings and qualities. But if we chant the mantra for 20 minutes each day for maybe 6 months, a year or even longer, then we start to rediscover what the mantra really is about.

When we are in harmony, we balance the heaven and earth energy within us. The harmony between heaven and earth is a very common theme within traditional Japanese spiritual teachings. Harmony between heaven and earth also indicates harmony between body and mind. Mikao Usui pointed this out within his precepts: *shinshin kaizen* – improve your heart/mind and body. Here he is pointing out that we need to harmonize our heart/mind and body. Or in other words we need to embody our spirituality. The word "embody" says it already: we need to be focused in our body to remember our True Self. If we are not in our body we become very ungrounded; how can we teach, communicate, and do our daily tasks if we are off with the fairies? If we think that a spiritual practice is about not being in our body, then we will have difficulty because we will be unable to embody the practice. Many people see a meditation practice as an escape from issues, or a way of ignoring them, but that is not real meditation. Real meditation is being fully in your body, while connected to heaven at the same time: thus in complete harmony. Again we see a link between the mantra and the precepts.

Each and every master, regardless of the era or the place, heard the call and attained harmony with heaven and earth.
– Morihei Ueshiba

To begin to get a glimpse of our True Self we need to first remember our embodiment of earth energy, and then we remember our embodiment with heavenly energy. This creates harmony. Our harmony was lost because we split up heaven and earth energy within us. This takes place due to our conditioning: our upbringing, what our parents told us, our education, seeing things as separate, etc. But the teachers of old, like Mikao Usui, knew that to remember our True Self, we need to harmonize the two opposite forces of heaven and earth energy within us again.

When this starts to happen we move into the state of mind of oneness, and slowly we get glimpses of our True Self. With more daily practice we start to then integrate this state of mind in all we do. In this way we are removing the last lampshades so that our True Self can shine in all its glory.

True Self is the Self that existed before the division of heaven and earth and before one's father and mother were born. This Self is the Self within me, the birds and the beasts, the grasses and the trees and all phenomena. It is exactly what is called "Buddha Nature".
– Takuan Soho, *The Unfettered Mind: Writings of the Zen Master to the Sword Master*

Conclusion

What will clear up all our emotional and mental issues all at once? Rediscovering our True Self. This is really the heart of Sei Heiki. Without rediscovering our True Self, we will be attached to and create new emotional and mental habits all the time. This means that we need to keep working with the mantra. If we understand where this signpost is pointing at, we can start to go straight to the root of all our emotional and mental issues. Why waste time that we do not have? We do not know when our end will be: it might be today or tomorrow. Better to start right at this moment by remembering our True Self. When we remember our True Self all our emotional and mental issues suddenly disappear. Our confused mind is like a room that is completely dark; when we suddenly switch on the light of our True Self, all the darkness disappears in one instant.

In Japan harmony has traditionally been greatly valued.
– H. E. Davey, *The Teachings of Tempu: Practical Meditation for Daily Life*

Chapter 12

Hon Sha Ze Sho Nen – I Am Right Mind

The third mantra within Mikao Usui's teachings also points towards our True Self and includes many insights about the qualities of our True Self.

The Meaning of the Mantra

In many modern teachings this mantra is used to help you with distance healing and therefore is only used when you do distance healing. But what was Mikao Usui's intent for using this mantra within his teachings? And was it really all about distance healing, or much more? Was it meant to be meditated upon, or chanted like the other mantras, to rediscover our True Self?

Hon 本 means true, book, origin, real, to find the origin in. In Buddhist tradition, Hon is often used in combination with other kanji to point to our original self or True Self, for example *honshin*, which means true mind or original mind.

Sha 者 means a person, someone, the one [who, which], he/she who is.

Ze 是 means right, correct, just so, this, justice, perfectly, it is this.

Sho 正 means correct, true, straight, the basis of correct knowledge, righteous.

Nen 念 means thought, feeling, mindfulness, mind, memory, meditative wisdom, patience, forbearance.

We could therefore say that Hon Sha Ze Sho Nen means: My original self/true self is a correct thought; I am right mindfulness, I am right mind; or Find the origin of your self in the true state of meditative wisdom.

The Right Mind is the mind that does not remain in one place.

It is the mind that stretches throughout the entire body and self. The Confused Mind is the mind that, thinking something over, congeals in one place.

– Takuan Soho, *The Unfettered Mind: Writings from a Zen Master to a Master Swordsman*

In looking at the translation of this mantra we can already see that it has nothing to do with distance healing. In fact the opposite is true; it is about rediscovering that there is no distance at all! It points straight to rediscovering our True Self.

To train with serious, esoteric, spiritual teachers in Japan, you either have to be invited by the teacher or to be recommended by one of the teacher's long-time students. I always wanted to train with an esoteric Japanese priest to understand what Mikao Usui himself was practicing and experiencing. This in turn would help me to teach Mikao Usui's teachings from a more traditional Japanese spiritual perspective. In 2012 I was finally introduced to Takeda Hakusai Ajari, who is the Deshi of Yusai Sakai Dai Ajari. Sakai Dai Ajari, who passed away in 2013, was a living treasure and Buddha in Japan. But before Takeda Hakusai allowed me to become his student he asked me many questions about Mikao Usui's teachings. He even did a Reiki course in Japan to see how the system of Reiki was taught there. He was very disappointed. For him Mikao Usui's teachings are all about rediscovering your True Self, which was not emphasized in the Japanese Reiki branches he investigated. One of the questions he asked me was what I thought 本者是正念 Hon Sha Ze Sho Nen was all about. I answered these questions as best as I could. He later told me that he was happy with my understanding of Mikao Usui's teachings and what the tools meant. He said that if I had answered the questions like he saw them explained in the branches of the system of Reiki that he investigated in Japan, he would not have invited me to become his student. When I finally trained with him in Japan for 7 days, one on one, he explained that 本者是正念 means, I am Right Mind. Right

Mind, he said, is a very important element to embody within yourself. Because it is only through this that we start to understand ourselves and what helping others really is about. I still hear some other words of his echoing through my mind: *Let's explore Mikao Usui's enlightenment together so that we might attain the same enlightenment as Mikao Usui.*

The Inner Teachings of Hon Sha Ze Sho Nen

So to where does this mantra within Mikao Usui's inner teachings really point? As I said before, it is pointing straight at our True Self. When we see ourselves as being here, and another person as being there, we create a distance; we are distancing ourselves from someone or something. The more we distance ourselves from someone, the harder it becomes to be compassionate towards him and to experience a unification and intimacy with him. Real compassion can only start to happen when we feel a deep sense of oneness and intimacy with others.

Right Mindfulness is about making sure our mind doesn't get carried away by labeling things. We normally label what we see, feel, hear, touch, or smell, either good or bad and then deal with it accordingly. However, when we have a direct experience of Right Mindfulness, we begin to stop labeling things. We just see things as they are, and we don't get carried away by our dualistic thinking. When we have an understanding of Right Mindfulness, we are not distracted by all the confused dualistic thoughts that come up. This is often called *munen*, no thought.

This poem reflects Right Thought:

In spring the flowers,
In autumn the moon,
In summer the breeze,
In winter the snow,
If in the serenity of the heart,
there is no attachment,

all seasons are well.

– Hui-K'ai

Mikao Usui put gems into his teachings to hint at what he was really trying to teach. We can only help others to find their non-dual nature if we have rediscovered it for ourselves. This is also why Level II is called Okuden, inner or hidden teachings: they help us to rediscover what is hidden within us. If we use the tools taught in Okuden Level II externally, we will have difficulty in getting the direct experience, but when we internalize them, we can gain a much deeper experience.

Shonen 正念 is part of the Buddha's teachings of the Eightfold Noble Path. Since Mikao Usui was a Buddhist practitioner, we should not be surprised to see traces of his own personal Buddhist journey in the system of Reiki.

The teachings of the Eightfold Noble Path are:

Right views
Right thoughts
Right speech
Right acts
Right living
Right effort
Right mindfulness
Right meditation

We could therefore also say that Hon Sha Ze Sho Nen is a person who has embodied the Eightfold Path.

In Sanskrit, the word for "right" is samma. It means "to go along with," "to go together," "to turn together." It originally comes from a term that means "to unite." So "right" is a state of being in which everything can live together, or turn together, united. Right is a state of human life in which we live in peace and harmony with all other beings. It is right, beyond our ideas of right or wrong, good or bad.

– Dainin Katagiri, *You Have to Say Something*

Within the kanji of Hon Sha Ze Sho Nen, 本者是正念, is also the kanji of Nen, 念, and within this we can also see the kanji of Shin/Kokoro, 心. Shin/Kokoro is called the radical of Nen; a radical is a clue to of the origin of the kanji and also to the general meaning. Shin/Kokoro means heart/mind, wholeheartedness, the enlightened mind, essence, and the mind as the principle of the universe, center and core. So again we can see that this mantra is pointing towards heart/mind and our True Self.

Quality

The quality of this mantra is interconnectedness or Oneness. If we look at the system of Reiki, the more practitioners gain a deeper direct understanding of right mindfulness by internalizing the mantras, the more they start to see that there is no distance, no past/present/future, just Oneness. It is the first step to experiencing non-duality; thus this mantra is already pointing towards the last mantra within Mikao Usui's teachings, Dai Kômyô, our innate great bright light. In fact all the mantras together form a path which we can walk upon; this is the path from not knowing our True Self to knowing our True Self.

As a human being, you have the profound desire to be free from suffering and know oneness. But real oneness is not something you can understand objectively; you must become one with it.

– Dainin Katagiri, *Each Moment Is the Universe*

Imagine that you are doing a hands-on healing session on someone, your client is lying or sitting down, you put your hands on him and you think you are channeling the energy through you. It comes from outside of you, through you and into the client. Now imagine that you, the client, and the universe are one and the same, oneness. When this oneness occurs, we have a much bigger potential because now all the boundaries have dropped away, there is no you, no client, just pure potential. This is the true quality of Hon Sha Ze Sho Nen.

Conclusion

By looking deeply into the mantras of Okuden Level II we start to rediscover what they are really about. Hon Sha Ze Sho Nen is all about remembering our oneness with the universe. Then we discover that there is no distance and also no time of past, present, and future. This state is where real deep healing starts to take place within ourselves. It is only when we start to have the direct experience of oneness that we rediscover real compassion. If we feel this oneness, then we need to be kind to ourselves, otherwise we will not be kind to others. In turn, we need to be kind to others or we are not kind to ourselves. At this stage of your practice, you also start to see what effect it has on the world when we do not come from this place of compassion. Thus to be of real help to the world, we need to start to embody this direct experience of oneness. This was the real message of Mikao Usui by utilizing this mantra within his teachings.

Additional Teachings

I have added this specific chapter to look at some additional teachings for this mantra. This is mainly due to the many questions I am often asked by existing practitioners and teachers about this specific mantra.

Distance Healing

I often get asked if it is good to "send" healing to the past or to the future. When we focus on the past or the future we are being taken out of this moment. The past is past, the future has not arrived, and even the present we cannot really find. So it is much better to stay focused on this moment.

> *The past is already past. Don't try to regain it.*
> *The present does not stay. Don't try to touch it.*
> *From moment to moment. The future has not come.*
> *Don't think about it beforehand.*
> – P'ang Yun, in Stephen Addiss, *Zen Sourcebook: Traditional Documents from China, Korea, and Japan*

The more we do our healing in this moment without judging if our past issues are bad or good, without judging future events, the more we start to be free from the grip of the three times. And when we are free, our innate great bright light starts to shine more and more. The three times are lampshades we have put over our innate great bright light, thus limiting ourselves. Just Be. This is easier said than done of course, but if we have our dedicated daily practice, we will get there; we will get glimpses of our True Self. This is what meditation with *hon sha ze sho nen* is trying to show us, but if we do not internalize this mantra then it will never show its face.

Past, present, and future are made by thinking. Original face has no past, no present, no future. We only have moment. Moment is yours – infinite time, infinite space. If you make this moment clear, then your whole life is clear, also next life clear. If this moment is not clear, then everything not clear.
– Seung Sahn, in "BOOM! An Interview with Zen Master Seung Sahn," *Tricycle Magazine*

If we heal ourselves in this moment then we are simultaneously healing our future and past issues. If we "send" healing to the future so that we get a job, for example, then that means we are worried that we will not get the job. Concentrating on the future is therefore based on worry and when we take the precepts to heart we have to let go of worry, which means we stay in the moment.

The word "sending" is another stumbling block, because as soon as we use that word, we are already in our confused mind. Sending means that you see yourself as separate from everything else, that you are here and the person you are sending to is over there. But it is only in our confused mind that we think we are separate; in our True Self we are always interconnected. This is the same with the word "distance." Distance means that we have distanced ourselves from someone, so how can we feel that we are interconnected with the other person?

As we go deeper into the heart of Mikao Usui's teachings we therefore also start to realize that there is no need to hold a photo, use your leg as a surrogate for the other person, or to pretend that your teddy bear is the other person, etc. All we have to do is to remember that we are already one, already interconnected with the other person. Now we have moved from doing distance healing and sending healing to Being Reiki. By Being Reiki we have the direct experience that we have always been one and interconnected.

Human consciousness can go anywhere in the universe in an instant. You must endeavor to develop your consciousness quickly and not rely on the symbols for too long.
– Note from a student of Mikao Usui from Hiroshi Doi's manual

Permission

Now we come to another interesting question which has been asked many times: Do we need to ask permission to do distance healing? By looking deeper into the real meaning of *hon sha ze sho nen* we start to discover that there is no need to ask permission. Remember, one of the metaphors Mikao Usui utilized in his teachings is being a great bright light. So imagine being the sun. Does the sun ask permission to shine? Of course not! The sun does not ask permission to shine, it just shines, and yet people take accordingly from the sun. Some like to lie in the sun all day, some want to sit in the sun during their lunch break, while others stay indoors enjoying its natural light. Each person takes what he or she needs from the sun, not what the sun thinks they should have. But here comes an important element: the sun doesn't think, "Now I am doing something, now this person needs to receive my rays and that person doesn't get anything." This is what we normally do; we make judgments as to what a person needs or does not need. However, our judgments are clouded by our own filters of anger, worry, and fear. Do we really know what another person needs? Think about this honestly. Most of the time we do not even know what we need for ourselves so how can we think we know what other people need?! Therefore, like the sun just shine, just Be.

When we just shine our great bright light into the world without any judgments, then the whole universe can take from us whatever they need. If someone doesn't want anything, fine; if someone wants something, fine too. Remember we are always interconnected anyway, so in that state we are always sharing.

All we have to do is remember that interconnectedness, set our intent that they receive whatever they need, and sit in that interconnected state of mind. Remember that the kanji for the precept kindness also means intimacy; *hon sha ze sho nen* helps us to become intimate with all that is, because only then can real kindness take place. Simple, but oh so difficult – why? Because we always want to do something. So again we need to move away from doing Reiki to Being Reiki.

Protection

To realize our state of mind of oneness, we need to let go of all our fears and therefore also from the need to protect ourselves. Many practitioners and teachers feel the need to protect themselves from other people's negative energy. This need for protection comes from our own confused minds in which we think we are separate and not one with everything. Of course if we look deeply we are separate and yet also one with everything. Both happen simultaneously.

The first question we need to ask ourselves is, why do we feel we need protection? The real answer is that we have fear: fear that we will pick up something unwanted from the client. We have this kind of fear within ourselves because we can't see the whole picture but only parts of it – we are not grounded, not centered, not realizing the truth. This fear makes us unstable, which also means that if we try to protect ourselves with, for example, the visualization of a bright light around us, then that visualization is based on fear, which in turn means it is unstable. We could call this kind of visualization "outer protection" as we see it external from ourselves. But what is fear? FEAR = False Evidence Appearing Real.

We experience fear because we cling to the "I."

- "I am getting your negative energy."
- "I am not feeling good after performing a hands-on healing

session."
- "I am picking up your physical issues."

All these statements have their base in a strong grasping of the "I." But who is this "I"? Normally we only relate to the relative "I," but when we go deeper into our personal practice we start to find our ultimate relation to the "I." This "I" and ego we cling to is false evidence appearing real.

> With no more ego there is nothing to fear.
> – Taisen Deshimaru, *Mushotoku Mind: The Heart of the Heart Sutra*

Let's now change our viewpoint for a moment. If we have to protect ourselves from taking on the client's "negative" energy, then what about our client?! Does the client also need to protect him/herself while lying on the table? Wouldn't the client also take on the practitioner's "negative" energy? Because if we have the fear that we will pick something up from our client then it can also be the other way around! Strangely, this doesn't seem to enter the practitioner's or teacher's mind. Why? It's because we only feel the need to protect ourselves. In other words, it is an ego trip, it is all about the "I."

Some teachers say, "Wash your hands after a hands-on healing session because you touched the client or worked in the client's energy field and now you might have taken on some of the client's 'negative' energy." This also implies that the client needs to wash him or herself after a treatment, as the client has also touched you! In response to this you might think, "No, my client only lies there. It was I who put my hands on the client." This comes once again from the ego, the "I." Just try it, put your hands on someone: okay it looks like you are touching the person because we associate touch with our hands, but the other person is touching your hands through their body! Right or not right?

Touch a tree, and now realize that the tree is also touching you; touch an animal and now you realize that the animal is also touching you – it is never a one-way street. We can touch with our whole being, our eyes, our hands, our skin, our energy, and don't forget the most important one: our mind. The whole idea of protection comes from our projection of grasping to the "I" – the practitioner considers him or herself as the doer and therefore can only pick stuff up, not the other way around. Our client is as much participating in the whole process as we are.

Fear comes from being worried and this brings us back to the precepts. We feel the need to protect ourselves because we worry that we will pick something up, that we will become contaminated with our client's stuff. But the precept says: "Do not worry!" So if we still feel the need to use an outer form of protection then this also means that we are not really grasping the precepts. This is why we first of all need to understand the precepts; without this our hands-on healing practice becomes unstable.

And what about the precept of compassion? What if you are doing a hands-on healing session on your client and afterwards your client says, "Please, can I give you all my issues? I've had enough of them." What would you say? If we were truly compassionate we would say, "Yes, of course. Let me take them from you, no problem." This is real compassion, taking on someone else's suffering. Taking on another person's pain and suffering is a wonderful way of helping to release our own fears and attachments and also to awaken pure compassion in ourselves. Even thinking about taking on another person's suffering will help us contemplate some of the other precepts, like worry and anger. So this practice/intent is a great antidote for our own pain and suffering. In needing to protect ourselves, we only strengthen our own fears and worries; we push ourselves away from real compassion as well. Often we are afraid to take on someone else's stuff as it brings up our own fears, anger, worry, you name it. A mother would have this kind of intent for her child; she would gladly take on the child's pain. When it comes to strangers we get scared.

Taking what is bad onto oneself and passing on what is good to others, and forgetting oneself and benefiting others – that is the height of compassion.
– Saicho, in Jiko Kohno, *Right View, Right Life: Insights of a Woman Buddhist Priest*

One other major issue is that we have fear because we are not properly grounded within our physical body. Remember the Weeble Wobbles? "Weebles wobble but they don't fall down!" Why do Weebles not fall? Because they have their weight at the bottom. Most of us, in our modern society, carry the weight in our head: too much TV, computers, intellectualizing, judging where to place the hands and what else to do during a treatment, mobile phone, you name it, it is all in the head. This makes us very unstable. We need to remember our center again, the *hara*, our foundation, and this can be done with the meditation practices taught within Mikao Usui's teachings which focus on the *hara* and the earth energy. The more we practice these kinds of meditation techniques, the more grounded we become. Like a Weeble Wobble, we might experience something during a hands-on healing session but we do not get scared or fearful, we do not fall over. Rather, we move straight back into our center. As our focus is directed inwards, into our *hara*, this is our "inner protection."

We are firmly protected from the inside. That is our spirit. We are protected from the inside, always, incessantly, so we do not expect any help from outside.
– Shunryu Suzuki, *Not Always So*

So we feel the need to protect ourselves because we fear that we might pick up "negative" energy from our client. But what is "negative" energy anyway? What one person might find negative, another might find positive. For example, you might do a hands-on healing session on someone and see lots of black stuff. You might get scared and label it negative, while someone else sees the same black stuff and it reminds her of a beautiful black night sky. This is the same experience, but a different kind of labeling. You might do a treatment on someone who has a cold and you get worried that you might pick it up, because you label the cold negative. Someone else does a hands-on healing on the same person but doesn't label the cold as negative, but just accepts it as it is. The latter practitioner is in a much better state of mind. Worry triggers imbalance within our own mind. This is why we need to clear the mind first before we can become stable practitioners and teachers. If our mind is unstable, our body and energy will also be unstable, and this means we are more vulnerable to being knocked over.

> The spiritual aspect of valor is evidenced by composure – calm presence of mind. Tranquility is courage in repose...A truly brave man is ever serene; he is never taken by surprise; nothing ruffles the equanimity of his spirit. In the heat of battle he remains cool; in the midst of catastrophes he keeps level his mind.
> – Nitobe Inazo, *Bushido: The Soul of the Samurai*

When we go deeper into the heart of the system of Reiki we start to realize that we are all interconnected in the first place. At a relative level we are separate, but at the ultimate level we are all interconnected. When we realize this interconnectedness we start to realize aspects of our True Self. This means that on this deeper level there is no giving or taking, no coming or going, no division between practitioner and client; there is just interconnectedness and that is all. This state of mind is the "ultimate protection." This means that within our personal practice we need to grow from "outer protection" to "inner protection" and then into "ultimate protection." This last kind of protection is the state of mind of I am Right Mind as symbolized by *hon sha ze sho nen*.

Here is an example I often demonstrate in class with a physical cardboard box, if available, which I put in front of me. When we feel the need to protect ourselves we create a wall between ourselves and our client, thus separating ourselves from the interconnectedness of our client and the universe. Imagine erecting a cardboard box which symbolizes our wall of protection. But as soon as there is a wall I can kick it, I can damage it – it is vulnerable. At this stage in the class I kick the cardboard box, and it flies here, there and everywhere. It gets hurt, it gets worried, and afterwards we need to fix the box, repair it – symbolizing repairing our own energy and mind, maybe by washing our hands, clearing our own energy from the "negativity" of our client after a hands-on healing session. But what if...I take the cardboard box and flatten it, making it completely open. Can I still kick it? No, there is nothing to kick! This openness, if it comes from the right place of course – our center, the *hara* – is the best protection. There is nothing to kick, nothing to damage, nothing to hurt. This open state of mind is the state of mind of *mushin*, "no-mind," the ultimate form of protection. This state of mind is like space, and we cannot hurt space; we can blow up walls, but we cannot blow up space. This kind of spaciousness is symbolized by the Dai Kômyô, the mantra taught within Shinpiden. Shinpiden means mystery teachings, and it is all about unlocking the mystery of how we relate to the universe and the universe relates to us. Or in other words these mystery teachings are about rediscovering our True Self, the ultimate protection.

Only through sincerity, through being open to accepting

things as they are in each situation, can one truly live each day as if it was one's whole life.

– Sakai Yusai, in Stephen G. Covell, "Learning to Preserve: The Popular Teachings of Tendai Ascetics", *Japanese Journal of Religious Studies*, Volume 31, number 3 (2004)

Chapter 13

Dai Kômyô

The traditional Japanese system of Reiki uses several symbols and mantras in its teachings and ongoing practices. These symbols and mantras are tools that help you deepen your understanding of and directly experience your True Self.

However, some of these symbols are not actually symbols. They are kanji, a Japanese system for writing words and ideas. Since these kanji are frequently displayed in Japanese temples, on Japanese statues, and in Japanese martial art schools, they are not exclusive to the system of Reiki. One of these kanji is Dai Kômyô, which is taught within Shinpiden Level III. In the last few years there has been some debate about Dai Kômyô, and whether Mikao Usui utilized it or not. As stated before, Hiroshi Doi knew of a student of Mikao Usui who was taught the Dai Kômyô by Mikao Usui himself. Mrs. Takata knew and taught the Dai Kômyô and so did Chujiro Hayashi who taught it to Mrs. Takata. However, some of Chujiro Hayashi's and Mikao Usui's students weren't taught the Dai Kômyô. Why? Because both Mikao Usui and Chujiro Hayashi taught their students according to their spiritual progress. So if the students weren't ready, why teach them something they were not ready for? This is why some students knew about it and others not.

Hiroshi Doi also has some notes from a student of Mikao Usui and one of these notes states: "Komyo exists in me and I exist in Komyo." This phrase is pointing towards Dai Kômyô. The great bright light exists in me and I exist in the great bright light. However, from a traditional Japanese viewpoint *kômyô* also stands for the light of the Buddha. Thus we could say: The light of the Buddha exists in me and I exist in the light of the Buddha. We can also see a link to this within the precept: This is the center of Buddhahood. This means that if we embody the precepts we are in the center of *kômyô*, now we have realized our great bright light, Dai Kômyô.

Does it really matter if some teachers knew it and some others did not? Most important is why is this mantra is taught within Mikao Usui's teachings and how to embody it! The mantra taught at this level is Dai Kômyô, 大光明, which means Great Bright Light. This is the light of Anshin Ritsumei, our True Self. By using this mantra, Mikao Usui was pointing out the very heart of his teachings: rediscovering our innate great bright light, our True Self.

The Meaning of the Mantra

Let's translate the kanji of Dai Kômyô:

大 Dai
光 Kô
明 Myô

Literally, the three kanji that comprise Dai Kômyô can be translated as:

Dai – large, great, big
Komyo – hope, glory, bright future
Kô – ray or light
Myô – bright, light, spell, mantra
Thus, a few ways that Dai Kômyô can be translated are:

• Great light spell
• Great light mantra
• Great bright light

The usual English translation is Great Bright Light. However, within certain esoteric Japanese spiritual traditions, these kanji represent the title for a 23-syllable Sanskrit mantra, in which case Dai Kômyô is sometimes written as Dai Kômyô Shingon and translated as Great Light Spell or Great Light Mantra.

In other Japanese esoteric traditions, Dai Kômyô is linked with Dainichi Nyorai, the Cosmic Buddha. According to the late Dento Dai Ajari Ryuko Oda of the Kyoasan School of Shingon Buddhism, Dainichi Nyorai personifies the essential nature of the universe and symbolizes the wisdom and compassion that allows you to realize the true nature of your mind. Within these traditions, Dai Kômyô is understood as a symbolic represen-tation of the universe's essence and our True Self. Embodying Dai Kômyô is also embodying emptiness (Jp. *ku*).

The Inner Teachings of Dai Kômyô

When looking closely at the kanji of Dai Kômyô, you can discover many different layers.

Dai – As previously noted, Dai can be translated as great, large, or big. But, in some Japanese esoteric schools, this kanji also represents the five elements (Jp. *goshiki*) of earth, water, fire, air, and space. Within these traditions, everything that exists is made up of the five elements. Among several Buddhist schools, a sixth element is often added to the five – the element of mind or consciousness. In these traditions, Dainichi Nyorai (Cosmic Buddha) is often portrayed with his hands in the Chiken-in mudra, the mudra of the six elements – earth, water, fire, air, space, and mind or consciousness. It is through the mind element that you understand the true nature of the other five elements; it is the lens through which you experience things you ordinarily consider to be outside yourself. Dai can also be interpreted as a human being standing tall and being great.

Kô – Superficially, the Kô kanji means light or ray. At a much deeper level, it represents your innate light, your True Self. This innate light has enormous healing potential, not only for you, but also for others. This is the light and wisdom of non-duality. To understand how this light functions, it may be useful to consider the light of the sun. The sun's rays shine on everything equally, without judgment. To accept the rays of the sun, you only need to stand in the sunlight. This is how the innate light of our True Self works – it shines everywhere; all we need do is stand in its light.

This kanji also stands for a fire on an altar, where the fire symbolizes purification. It is only through purification that we can rediscover the light within ourselves.

Subhakarasimha states this in his Commentary on the Mahavairocana Sutra about why Mahavairocana (Dainichi Nyorai) is called the Great Light:

It eliminates darkness and illuminates all things;
It enables the fulfilment of all works;
It is the light which is neither created nor destroyed.

Myô – The third kanji, Myô, is actually made up of two separate kanji. The kanji on the left represents the sun, while the kanji on the right represents the moon. In many Japanese esoteric teachings, the sun represents the female aspect of wisdom (Jp. *chie*), while the moon represents the male aspect of compassion (Jp. *jihi*) and/or method (Jp. *hoben*). Both these qualities emerge as a result of deepening your spiritual practice. Wisdom and compassion/method are not separate entities, but intertwined with each other. One cannot exist without the other. When the sun and moon are together in the night sky it is very bright; this brightness is also symbolic for clarity in your mind.

The great Bodhisattvas wear on their heads a jeweled crown of the Five Wisdoms as well as that wisdom which is like the sun and moon and illuminates the various dark recesses of the mind.

– Holy Fudo Myo-o Secret Darani Sutra

The sun and moon kanji that comprise the Myô kanji thus give the Dai Kômyô a much deeper meaning than simply Great Light Mantra or Great Bright Light. The sun and moon combined together into one symbol represent the union of absolute truth (Jp. *kutai*) and relative truth (Jp. *ketai*). In the Mahayana Buddhist traditions, kutai is the truth of emptiness, while ketai is the truth of temporariness. The union of kutai and ketai is the truth of the middle way (Jp. *chutai*), which is the truth that all things are dependently originated, neither arising nor ceasing. The three truths of ketai, kutai, and chetai are central concepts in Tendai Buddhist teachings and practices. In fact, through deepening meditation practices, Tendai practitioners can directly experience a unification of the three truths in a single mind (Jp. *enyu no sangan*). This state of mind is called "the three truths of wisdom in a single mind" (Jp. *isshin sanchi*).

Putting all this together, the true meaning of Dai Kômyô is really a spiritual experience of your own True Self. It therefore doesn't just mean great bright light, but also stands for emptiness and non-duality.

In certain Japanese esoteric traditions, it's common to recite just the title of a mantra or sutra, rather than the entire text. This is based on the view that the title embodies the whole. For example, in Nichiren Buddhism, there is a practice whereby one chants the title of the Lotus Sutra (Jp. *Hoke-kyo*), which is Namu Myoho-Renge-Kyho. This type of practice also applies to Dai Kômyô. However, in this case the Great Light Mantra is not the Dai Kômyô mantra used within the system of Reiki. Instead, Dai Kômyô (sometimes called Dai Kômyô Shingon) is the title of a specific 23-syllable Sanskrit mantra: *On abokya beiroshanō makabodara mani handoma jimbara harabaritaya un.*

When chanted, the practitioner often visualizes the 23 syllables as a wheel.

The essential characteristic of this practice is purification – you call upon the Great Purifying Light of the universe in order to remember your own inner Great Bright Light and experience complete unification with the universe.

According to Dr. Henny van Der Veere, a Shingon priest who teaches at the Centre of Japanese Studies of the University of Leiden in Holland, this mantra was originally non-sectarian and only later included within different Japanese esoteric teachings. Today, however, Dai Kômyô is utilized in Tendai, Mikkyo, Shingon, Shinto, and Shugendo. For example, in the esoteric Japanese Buddhist path known as Shugen Mikkyo (a form of Shugendo) there are two ways this mantra is used. The first is where you recite the mantra to overcome inner obstructions such as worry, fear, or attachments. The second is where you recite the mantra 100 or 1000 times in order to "guide" the soul of a dead person. Through this latter practice (Jp. *eko gongyo shiki*), you are able to transfer merit to others.

Dai Kômyô is also used in a text of the Mikkyo tradition of Tendai called *komyo ku*. This is practiced in *juhachi-do*, a traditional Mikkyo style that is common to all esoteric ritual patterns. In the komyo ku, you merge with the "Light Wisdom" of the Original Buddha Nature (Dainichi Nyorai). This manifests as the pure light of your radiant self, a natural energetic force.

In Shingon Buddhism, the Great Light Mantra is chanted for purification of past actions, either for yourself or others. In Mark Unno's book *Shingon Refractions: Myoe and the Mantra of Light* it states:

The Sutra of the Mantra of Light of the Baptism of Vairocana of the Unfailing Rope Snare says: If sentient beings attain this baptism and mantra anywhere so that it reaches their ears just two, three, or seven times, then all evil hindrances will be eliminated. If one sits before the stricken for one, two, or three days and intones this mantra one thousand and eighty times every day with a full voice, then the hindrances of illnesses from past karma will be destroyed. Myoe used the mantra in several ways: in the complex rituals of a deity yoga, through which the mystic powers of the buddhas and bodhisattvas entered into the practitioner; in funeral rites; in the preparation of sand for alleviating karmic suffering, both physical and mental, in this life and the next; and in simple recitations as part of the daily monastic regimen of Kozanji where Myoe served as abbot.

In many Japanese martial arts (Jp. *budō*), a specific mantra – Shikin Haramitsu Dai Kômyô – is used at the start and end of each practice session. It is said that this mantra reflects both Buddhist and Shinto perspectives and is derived from an 8th-century Buddhist prayer. There are many ways to translate this mantra. One way is this: "If your whole heart has perfected the six perfections then you will realize enlightenment." These perfections are the six paramitas of Mahayana Buddhism: generosity, ethical behavior, patience, perseverance, concentration, and wisdom.

In the mid-19th century, several new religions (Jp. *shinshūkyō*) emerged in Japan, including Tenrikyo, Kurozumikyo, Oomoto kyo, Johrei, and the Soka Gakkai. Many of them utilized the Dai Kômyô for spiritual development and insight. Within the Johrei tradition, Mokichi Okada (1882–1955) taught people about the divine light of Johrei, which is not only a healing practice but also a way of life. On many Johrei shrines there is a scroll with the kanji of Dai Kômyô Shin Shin. This kanji of Dai Kômyô was used as a focus tool for healing and spiritual development. Before he started Johrei, Okada was involved in the spiritual teachings of Oomoto Kyo, which is said to have also used

Dai Kômyô.

Many of these new religions also took elements of Shugendo to aid them in their teachings and practices, and it is in Shugendo that you also find the Dai Kômyô. Professor Miyake Hitoshi states in his article "Religious Rituals in Shugendo": "It can also be said that shugendo provided the central model for the religious activities of many of the 'new' religions (e.g sectarian Shinto) that proliferated from the latter part of the nineteenth century and continue today."

Quality

The quality of Dai Kômyô is empowerment. But the word "empowerment" has brought a lot of confusion in the modern system of Reiki because it started to be only utilized during an "empowerment" which in turn is a *reiju*/initiation/attunement. Or in other words it became externalized. The quality of empowerment Mikao Usui had in mind was self-empowerment. We can only empower someone else if we have found that empowerment within ourselves. I cannot give you a cup of tea if I do not have a cup of tea myself! Dai Kômyô is therefore a mantra like the previous ones. By reciting this mantra for thousands of times we reach a state of self-empowerment. But, and here is the catch, for this mantra to be successful we need to have prepared our heart/mind and energy. Without this preparation, for most of us, the mantra will not lead to empowerment. We therefore need to first work with the previous meditation practices so that we have created a solid foundation to embody this kind of self-empowerment.

As mentioned before, this is one of the reasons Mikao Usui and Chujiro Hayashi only taught Dai Kômyô to those who had prepared themselves on a spiritual level.

Just get the root, don't worry about the branches, for someday you will come to have them naturally. If you have not attained the basis, even if you consciously study you cannot attain the outgrowths either.

– Zen Master Yangshan, in Thomas Cleary, *Zen Essence: The Science of Freedom*

Real empowerment comes from rediscovering our True Self; this is also when we receive the blessing of the universe: real *reiju*/initiation/attunement without the need for a person to perform a ritual on or for us. This is just like Mikao Usui experienced when he performed his meditation practice on Mt. Kurama for 21 days.

Conclusion

As noted above, in esoteric traditions, the fundamental essence of Dai Kômyô is its refining, cleansing quality. Within the traditional system of Reiki, Dai Kômyô is a centuries-old tool that makes an enlightened state of being accessible to modern practitioners. Working with Dai Kômyô, you consciously and repeatedly open yourself to the Great Bright Light of primordial, original enlightenment, so as to eventually experience your own transformation into that Great Bright Light – remembering our True Self.

This means that Dai Kômyô is nothing different than the precepts and the word Reiki. Reiki means our True Self, Dai Kômyô is our True Self symbolized as a great bright light, and the precepts are an intellectual description of our True Self. Mikao Usui put lots of signposts in his teachings, but they all point towards the same thing: rediscovering our True Self. Don't get distracted that there are many different signposts, as they are all pointing to the same place.

We can use the words "true self-confidence" in place of "enlightenment." True self-confidence means confidence in the true self, and confidence in the true self is a necessary requisite to happiness.

– Soko Morinaga, *Novice to Master: An Ongoing Lesson in the Extent of My Own Stupidity*

When we have embodied Dai Kômyô, we have internalized the precepts, we have become Reiki, and we have realized our True Self: this is empowerment.

Additional Teachings

I have added some additional teachings to this section to help you to gain a more direct experience of the Dai Kômyô.

Heart Sutra and Dai Kômyô

One of the most popular sutras within Japan is the Heart Sutra – Hannya Shingyo. This sutra is practiced in all major Japanese spiritual traditions, and I would therefore not be surprised if Mikao Usui had utilized this sutra himself. If we look deeply into his teachings, we see many links to the embodiment of the Heart Sutra. One of them is Dai Kômyô. If we embody Dai Kômyô we embody the precepts but also the Heart Sutra. Both of them point towards emptiness, non-duality, and our True Self. The quality of our True Self is emptiness (*ku* in Japanese) and non-duality; we cannot separate them, just as we cannot separate wetness from water.

> To abandon the ego is very difficult. It is only within ku, in infinite nothingness, in the total abandonment of the self, that the highest realization can be found. To understand this is to have satori.
> – Taisen Deshimaru, *Mushotoku Mind: The Heart of the Heart Sutra*

Mikao Usui's teachings are all about *anshin ritsumei*, satori, finding our True Self, the embodiment of Dai Kômyô. This is also why Mikao Usui used the word Reiki – the ki in Reiki is the same as *ku* – emptiness, which is the same as embodying Dai Kômyô. Again we can see how the inner heart of Mikao Usui's teachings always points towards the same place: remembering our True Self.

In Buddhism, this vital force is called ki: it is the essential constituent of the whole cosmos, and thus is equivalent to ku.
– Taisen Deshimaru, *Mushotoku Mind: The Heart of the Heart Sutra*

My teacher Takeda Hyakusai keeps saying, "Embody the Heart Sutra and you will understand Mikao Usui's teachings." However, one of the most important elements to remember is not just to memorize the Heart Sutra or know its meaning intellectually, but to embody it. How do we embody something? To embody the Heart Sutra or Dai Kômyô we need to sit on our butt and chant, do the meditation practices, and open our heart/mind, so that we can have the direct experience. Many serious teachers in Japan tell us to burn the sutras and to go into the mountains instead so that we can have this direct experience. This is like Mikao Usui who went into the mountains so that he too could remember his True Self.

The essential theme of the Hannya Shingyo is therefore the philosophy of ku.
– Taisen Deshimaru, *Mushotoku Mind: The Heart of the Heart Sutra*

To Die Once

Dai Kômyô is also interlinked with Mikao Usui's experience on Mt. Kurama.

It is said that when he asked his teacher about his spiritual progress, his teacher said, "You have to die once." So he took this advice and sat on Mt. Kurama for 21 days to meditate to die once. Some people suggest that he meant to physically die, but if that were the case it would have been much easier for him to climb Mt. Kurama and jump off a cliff, rather than to sit for a difficult practice for 21 days.

But if it was not the physical death that his teacher pointed to, what kind of death was it then? In Japanese spiritual traditions "to die once" means to go through the Great Death (Jp. *Daishi*) so that we are able to rediscover our True Self.

Mikao Usui's memorial stone states, "One day, he climbed kurama yama and after 21 days of a severe discipline without eating, he suddenly felt One Great Reiki over his head and attained enlightenment and he obtained Reiki Ryôhô." The purpose of this "severe discipline" was to help him "die once" so that he could rediscover his True Self. It was this Great Death experience that preceded his creation of the spiritual system of Reiki. It was after this experience that he really found purpose in his life and started to teach more and more people his spiritual teachings.

Is it possible to really live our lives fully without ever looking hard at death? I do not believe it is. Without staring death in the eye, as the perpetual reverse side of life, we cannot live life fully and completely.

– Soko Morinaga, *Novice to Master: An Ongoing Lesson in the Extent of My Own Stupidity*

It is possible that Mikao Usui was practicing Shugendo. Within Shugendo there is a very specific 21-day mountain practice in which you abstain from eating (in Japanese, *danjiki*) and drinking (in Japanese, *mizudachi*). This practice is suitable only for the rare, dedicated and prepared practitioner, called 餌食水无 読誦 修行 / だんじき みず なし どくじゅ しゅぎょう – *Danjiki-Mizunachi dokuju Shûgyô*. One of my teachers, Rev. Kûban Jakkôin, has done this specific 21-day Shugendo practice. This is one of the reasons I train with these kinds of teachers, so that I can understand what Mikao Usui was doing himself so that I can share his ideas, insights and practices within the wider Reiki community.

What is even more interesting is that during this particular

21-day practice the practitioner focuses also on the deity Myoken Bosatsu. Myoken Bosatsu is linked to Mikao Usui's family. We can see this by looking at Mikao Usui's family crest, the Chiba Mon. Did Usui-san choose this particular practice because of his family heritage? Myoken Bosatsu is also related to having certain healing qualities and holds a sun and moon in her hands. Healing is a part within the system of Reiki and we can also see the sun and moon in Dai Kômyô.

The whole universe shatters into a hundred pieces.
In the great death there is no heaven and earth
Once body and mind have turned over
there is only this to say:
Past mind cannot be grasped,
present mind cannot be grasped,
future mind cannot be grasped.
– Dogen

The state of mind Dogen refers to is called the Great Death because it is the death of the ego, the death of the "I." If we want to take our spiritual practice deeper, then one day we need to go through the process of letting go of the "I," because it is only at that stage that we can rediscover our True Self. When we let go of the "I," of our dualistic life of separateness and suffering, we start to find the meaning of life: a life full of compassion and wisdom, a life of interconnectedness and harmony, a life full of light and inner joy.

For many years before his Mt. Kurama experience, Mikao Usui sought *anshin ritsumei*: enlightenment or satori. He finally realized that to attain this goal he needed to go through the Great Death experience, because it is only after going through the Great Death that *anshin ritsumei* will show its face. Therefore we could say that the Great Death is the gate through which we enter the state of mind of enlightenment. This state of mind is all about realizing non-duality, which is the ultimate reality.

Hakuin suggests that satori is necessarily preceded by "great doubt" (daigi) and "great death" (daishi). The practitioner has to be able and willing to let go of all securities and beliefs and throw himself or herself into the abyss of emptiness. Hakuin urges the practitioner to abandon all discriminating thoughts, to form the "ball of doubt" (gidan), and to penetrate the One Mind. This, Hakuin says, is the experience of "great death".
– Ninian Smart, *World Philosophies*

After experiencing this One Mind on Mt. Kurama, Mikao Usui created a system of teachings to help others also find the way to experience the Great Death. We can see that he was pointing out the Great Death in his teachings, for example within the precepts and the symbols and mantras. It is only when we have let go of the "I" that we can truly embody the precepts. Because it is the "I" who gets angry and worried, it is the "I" who gets in the way of being humble, honest, and compassionate. Thus the precepts are pointing towards Mikao Usui's own enlightened experience, the Great Death. So actually this Great Death is about gratitude for life, to live life at its fullest, because when we have let go of our biggest worry, fear of death, we are free: free to dance through life. It is at this stage that we really start to transform our lives and those of others.

Mikao Usui also showed some of his students the Dai Kômyô, which stands for the great bright light of *anshin ritsumei*, again pointing towards the Great Death. He included all these pointers in his teachings because it is only after the Great Death that we truly become alive. The following quotes powerfully illustrate the transformation into our True Self:

After several days in his [Hakuin] condition, which he also

later designated as the "Great Death" and interpreted as the dying of the ego and illusion [he] recounted how he "chanced to hear the sound of the temple bell and...was suddenly transformed. It was as if a sheet of ice had been smashed or a jade tower had fallen with a crash. Suddenly I returned to my senses...All my former doubts vanished as though ice had melted away. In a loud voice I called: 'Wonderful! Wonderful!'"
– Conrad Hyers, *Once-Born, Twice-Born Zen: The Soto and Rinzai Schools of Japan*

Suddenly, under some impetus unknown to me, the fog lifted and vanished. And it is not that the pain in my own body disappeared, but rather that the body that is supposed to feel the pain disappeared. Everything was utterly clear. Even in the dimly lit darkness, things could be seen in a fine clarity. The faintest sound could be heard distinctly, but the hearing self was not there. This was, I believe, to die while alive.
– Soko Morinaga, *Novice to Master: An Ongoing Lesson in the Extent of My Own Stupidity*

Mikao Usui was only able to create the system of Reiki after going through the Great Death experience because it was only then that he had the clarity, wisdom, and compassion to formulate what he had been looking for himself in some sort of teaching. These teachings are the legacy of his own satori and by practicing the system of Reiki as a spiritual practice we are stepping into the footsteps of Mikao Usui, so that one day we can go through the same gate of the Great Death that Mikao Usui went through.

I cannot stress enough that the ultimate goal of religion, whether we call it satori or peace of mind, is for each individual to live in peace and tranquility, to live a full and satisfying life.

– Soko Morinaga, *Novice to Master: An Ongoing Lesson in the Extent of My Own Stupidity*

Chapter 14

An Overview of Japanese
Esoteric Traditions

To better understand the Japanese esoteric traditions mentioned in the previous chapter, let's have a closer look at them. Rev. Kûban Jakkôin provided me with the following information for this book.

Tendai is based on Vajrayana and Mahayana Buddhist teachings. Saicho brought the teaching from China at the beginning of the Heian period, 1100 years ago. Their main text is the Lotus Sutra and their main temple is Enrykuji temple at Mt. Hiei, northeast of Kyoto. Several Buddhist schools stem from Tendai, including Pure Land and Nichiren.

Shingon, a form of Vajrayana Buddhism of the True Word, was brought by Kukai from China at the beginning of the Heian period, 1100 years ago. The Shingon doctrine is based on the Mahavairocana sutra (Jp. *Dainichi-kyo*) and the tantra of Sanmitsu-yuga, the Yoga of Triple Mysteries (the union between mantra [speech], mudra [action] and mandala [mind]). Unlike Tendai, Shingon was not a birth ground for other Buddhist sects. However, different Shingon sects were established after Kukai's death, including New Shingon (*shin-shingon*) of Buzan-ha, and Chizan-ha (started by the monk Kakuban). The Old Shingon (*kogi-shingon*) tradition is practiced inside the Koya san, Daigoji, Daikakuji, and Toji temples in Kyoto.

Shugendo is a set of vigorous practices for developing Siddhi (inner power). It was founded in Japan, 1300 years ago, by Enno Gyoja. As a tantric-based mountain practice that mixes Daoism and Shintoism (shamanism), it views the mountain as the perfect three-dimensional womb and diamond mandala of Dainichi

Nyorai (the Cosmic Buddha). According to Miyake Hitoshi, in his book *Shugendo: Essays on the Structure of Japanese Folk Religion*:

> At the beginning of the world there existed a state of undifferentiated chaos resembling a chicken egg, but it was filled with the sacred letter "A" of Dainichi Nyorai. Soon there separated from this both heaven and earth, and also the cosmic dual forces, yin and yang. Through the union of heaven and earth all things were born and, through the interaction of the cosmic dual forces, humans came into being.

Shugendo involves many prolonged ascetic practices that take place in natural settings over a period of 21, 100, or even 1000 days. Some Shugendo sects follow either Tendai or Shingon traditions.

Mikkyo, which means secret or deep understanding of Buddhist teachings, consists of three teachings:

* Tômitsu (pure esoteric teachings), the secret teaching of Shingon Buddhism
* Taimitsu (Tendai esoteric teachings), the secret teachings of Tendai Buddhism (divided into Sanmon mikkyo at the Enryakuji temple and Jimon mikkyo at the Onjoji/Miedera temple)
* Zômitsu (mixed esoteric teachings), the secret teaching of Shugen Buddhism.

Part IV

Reiju and Your True Self

Chapter 15

Reiju

The traditional Japanese word used by Mikao Usui for the initiation or attunement is Reiju.

> Over the course of the medieval period, secret initiation and lineal transmission became common practice in all schools of Buddhism, including the "new" Zen and Pure Land traditions, as well as in Shugendo (mountain ascetism), Onmyodo (yin-yang divination), and in Yoshida Shinto. The practice of secret transmission also developed in the cultural arts, including poetry, calligraphy, the No drama, biwa recitation, flower-arranging, tea ceremony; in the martial arts; and in the crafts and manufacturing arts. In short, this became the normative mode of transmitting knowledge in premodern Japan.
> – Jacqueline Stone, *Original Enlightenment and the Transformation of Medieval Japanese Buddhism*

The word Reiju can be translated as spiritual blessing or spiritual offering. The practice of Reiju has created a lot of confusion within the modern Reiki community, so let's see if we can clarify this a little.

First of all, as the translation indicates, a Reiju is spiritual in nature; it's not physical. Traditional teachings indicate that when Mikao Usui initially offered a Reiju to his students, there was no physical ritual. Instead, he was "just sitting" opposite the student. But this wasn't just any sitting – Mikao Usui was a living embodiment of the great bright light, Dainichi Nyorai, his True Self. This state of mind represents non-attachment, including non-attachment to our ego. It denotes a state of being without any sense of a "you" or an "I" or even of "doing." It epitomizes a space of open possibility. Mikao Usui was "just sitting" as the great bright light, encompassing the entire cosmos and being that space of open possibility.

In that space, Mikao Usui could offer the Reiju as a healing, a blessing, an initiation, or all at the same time. In that space, the student could receive whatever he or she needed, at that moment in time. There was no need for ritual, only the ability of the person "giving" the Reiju to be the great bright light. In Japanese, the essence of this state of being is called *nyu ga ga nyu*, or mind-to-mind transmission. Another translation of *nyu ga ga nyu* means, "self entering the Buddha and the Buddha entering the self." In other words, we could say that this kind of Reiju is from True Self to True Self, no separation. This is when both the teacher and student break that glass jar we discussed in the first chapter of this book. Both mingling together, non-duality, no division of "I" and "you," just Be.

The last, "initiation based on mind" (ishin kanjo), uses no form or ritual, and is considered the highest kind of initiation.
– Taiko Yamasaki, *Shingon Japanese Esoteric Buddhism*

If we really think that the Reiju is just a physical ritual, then we are not being honest – anyone can learn to do the physical ritual, but does this mean that they can offer a Reiju, a spiritual blessing, in a state of "being the great bright light"? If so, we should teach everyone in the world how to do the ritual, then we can all perform it on each other and within no time the world will be a better place.

Unfortunately, few modern Reiki teachers are able to facilitate the egoless, mind-to-mind transmission that is the foundation of Reiju. Many might even find it hard to understand the concepts, let alone "be" the great bright light. It is extremely difficult to completely step out of the way – our ego has such a strong grip on everything. This is why the system of Reiki is a spiritual and lifelong practice.

Even some of Mikao Usui's Shinpiden students had difficulty with being in this egoless state. Therefore, he borrowed a physical ritual designed to help his students remember their True Self. This borrowed ritual didn't have any symbols or mantras, only specific hand positions performed on the person receiving the Reiju. This specific ritual resembles many other initiation practices taught within Japanese esoteric traditions, like *kaji* for example. The symbols and mantras were added later, by Chujiro Hayashi, who studied with Mikao Usui during the last 10 months of Usui's life. Hayashi's intention, like that of Mikao Usui, was to help students remember their True Self. He viewed the symbols and mantras as spiritual keys, meant to unlock that which is hidden within.

> The basic 12 hand positions and the attunements procedures [with the symbols and mantras] we use today are all derived from Hayashi-sensei's techniques.
> – Hiroshi Doi, *A Modern Reiki Method for Healing*

When Hayashi taught the system of Reiki to Mrs. Takata, she referred to Reiju as an initiation, as evidenced in her personal diary. She saw the initiation as an opportunity for the student to have an initial experience that he or she is Reiki. As Mrs. Takata states in her dairy, "Let the true energy come out from within. It lies in the bottom of the stomach about 2 inches below the navel." There is no indication that Mrs. Takata ever referred to the Reiju as an attunement. However, after she died, some of her students – now teachers in their own right – started calling the initiation an attunement. And this is the term now in use in many countries and among many teachers.

Unfortunately, calling the Reiju an attunement gives rise to many misconceptions. One such misconception is that Reiki is external to the recipient. For example, some Reiki teachers say, "Without an attunement, you cannot channel Reiki." Others say, "An attunement is the transfer of the ability to channel Reiki, passed from a teacher to a student." Such statements contradict the teachings of Mikao Usui, since he taught that Reiki is our True Self, hidden within us, waiting to be rediscovered. It doesn't need to be "channeled" – which the Merriam-Webster dictionary defines as express, move, or carry – because it's already channeling within, through, and around us. For the same reason, it also doesn't need to be transferred from a teacher to a student. If either statement were actually true, then anyone who wasn't attuned would not be alive. Obviously, that is not the case!

To really understand the concept of what a Reiju is, we need to not only look at the cultural context within which Mikao Usui practiced Reiju – that is, as a spiritual blessing or offering as the great bright light – but also the practice tools that are taught within the system of Reiki. When we learn the Reiju within Shinpiden Reiki Level III, we are also taught the Dai Kômyô. By this time we should have a deep understanding of the precepts. Therefore, when we offer a Reiju we need to come from the state of mind of the precepts and the Dai Kômyô; both are in fact the same. Embodying the precepts means we embody Dai Kômyô, which means we have rediscovered our True Self.

Chapter 16

The Inner Heart of Reiju

The inner heart of Reiju is all about rediscovering our True Self or in other words rediscovering Reiki.

Let's ask ourselves: What is the most compassionate and profound Reiju? This would be if during this Reiju the student rediscovered her True Self in all its glory, and the teacher rediscovered her True Self in all its glory. Also, if this rediscovery of their True Self lasted their whole lifetime. But this is not that easy because for this to take place, the teacher needs to have a very solid practice in which she has removed enough lampshades that a big part of her True Self shines through. However, that is not enough either: the student needs to have done the same; both need to be perfectly ready and ripe. Even if both the teacher and student are ripe there also needs to be a certain trust and intimacy between them both for both "I's" – egos – to fall away at the same time. As this is most often not the case, the Reiju needs to be done again and again and again until one day both the teacher and student rediscover the True Self, and all lampshades are gone. This is also why practicing the system of Reiki as a spiritual practice is a lifelong journey.

As an alternative word for Reiju, rather than attunement, I prefer to say initiation, as that indicates an "initial" experience. During the Reiju the student will have an initial experience of the True Self. How brief or profound this experience is doesn't matter. This initial experience is like a seed, not planted by the teacher, but rediscovered by the student deep within herself. For a seed to grow we need to water it, hence the rain of Rei. The seed also needs heat and coolness to mature, hence the fire of Ki, and the sun and moon of Dai Kômyô. It also needs space, hence the spaciousness of our state of mind if we let go of anger, worry, if we are more true to our way and our True Self, and more compassionate to ourselves and others. The heat and spaciousness is also created by meditating on the symbols and mantras and practices like *joshin kokyu hō*. Or in simple words, Reiju helps us to gain an initial experience which is like a seed and by practicing the system of Reiki we bring the seed to fruition until one day it blossoms into rediscovering our True Self.

Here is another metaphor I like to use: Reiju is like pointing to the sliver of the waxing moon; we see a small part of it but not yet the whole. After the Reiju, which points out the sliver of the moon, we still need to keep practicing. Practicing with the tools provided by Mikao Usui: meditating on the precepts, doing the meditation practices, meditating on the symbols and mantras, practicing the moving meditation of hands-on healing, and being in the meditative state of Reiju. After lots of meditation practice we start to see the brightness of the full moon, our True Self. Reiju is just the first part, the pointing out of our True Self; the real remembering of our True Self needs to come through our own personal meditation practice.

Sometimes during or after a Reiju, people can become distracted by the colors or visions they experience. It's important to remember that these visions are not the real aim of Reiju. I like to joke with my students that it is very easy to see visions, like stars. For example during a Reiju, just hit your student on the head and they will see stars for days! It is also very easy to feel energy during a Reiju: just plug your student into the electrical outlet and they will feel energy.

Focusing our thoughts on feeling energy, hot hands, or seeing visions is just a trap of our confused mind. Rather than physical or psychic experiences during Reiju, the real aim should be the embodiment of the precepts in all that we do. Of course it is much easier to see stars or feel energy, and this is why many people would rather focus on these experiences than on the precepts, the inner heart of the teachings. In addition, if the teacher doesn't embody the precepts, how can he facilitate that space for his students? I cannot give you tea if I do not have tea. Thus we can also say that the inner heart of the Reiju is a direct experience of the precepts. If we are distracted by the need to see, feel, hear, smell, sense, and see things during a Reiju, we are moving away from a spiritual blessing into a mundane kind of blessing. A real spiritual blessing is connected to our heart/mind, our True Self.

For a Reiju to become a spiritual blessing, we also need to be balanced in mind, body, and speech. The teacher's mind needs to be One with the precepts, her body needs to be open and fluid, and her energy needs to be like a calm lake. The student's mind, body, and energy needs to also be in that same kind of state. During Reiju we will also use our intent (our mind) that the student receives whatever she needs. Our body will perform the physical ritual. And with our speech (energy), we can give a verbal instruction to the student to help her set her intent, that she receives whatever she needs. This also engages her mind. Her body needs to be not slouched but straight and open. And her energy needs to be as much as possible like a calm lake. Now the student's mind, body, and energy are involved, which means we have a possibility of merging with the mind, body, and energy of the universe.

Why did I use the image of a calm lake in the above discussion? The image of the lake is yet another metaphor for a Reiju. A calm lake is like a mirror and a mirror can reflect everything. However, a mirror doesn't judge or label, it just reflects. Therefore we can also see the Reiju as the teacher holding up a perfectly clear mirror so that the student can see his own True Self. In order for the teacher's mirror to be clear, he needs to practice and delve deep into the heart of the teachings; otherwise the mirror becomes a judging or labeling mirror. The student needs to look clearly into the mirror, or he will also start to judge and label. If Reiju allows us to glimpse our True Self, then we can remember it again and again in our daily life. The more we remember it, the more we will embody our True Self.

Chapter 17

Heritage of Reiju

Reiju is not unique to Mikao Usui's teachings and we can see many similarities with other initiations within Japanese esoteric traditions. The first kanji of Reiju is Rei 霊 which also symbolizes rain; we will discuss this in more detail in the next chapter. Rain or water is a very important element in the initiation teachings in Japan. The old Sanskrit name of initiation is Abhisheka; this word is sometimes still used by the older teachers and in old manuals in Japan. The Japanese name for Abhisheka is 灌頂 kanjo and stands for pouring from the peak, sprinkling water on the crown, and a ceremony to bestow mystic teachings.

> I was then given the fivefold abhisheka and received instruction into the grace of the Three Mysteries [sanmitsu].
> – Kukai, in Richard Bowring, *The Religious Traditions in Japan*

As we can see, the imagery of both Reiju and Abhisheka is exactly the same; within Reiju, spiritual rain pours over the student's and teacher's heads. Of course we can also see the first kanji of Reiju in Reiki. All of these aspects help us to understand Usui's teachings better, which in turn will help us to gain a clearer perspective of the journey to rediscovering our True Self. Sometimes these rituals were very physical and other times it was just mind-to-mind (Jp. *Ishin kanjo*) with no physical ritual or visualization. This would of course depend first of all on the teacher, but also on the student. If the student needed a more physical aspect for support, then even if the teacher could perform a mind-to-mind initiation, it would have been of no use as the student was not ready. But of course the teacher could only perform a mind-to-mind initiation if he or she had rediscovered a very big part of his or her True Self. It is said that Mikao Usui would just sit opposite his students and perform the mind-to-mind initiation.

> There is a profound initiation which is performed in all the esoteric Buddhist and Shugen teachings; it is an initiation by heart/mind called: Ishin Kanjo. This initiation can be achieved anywhere, without any material required. It is an initiation which is apart from space and of time, in a place that only the Buddhas know following intense ascetic periods for the practitioner. More important than a simple initiation, this initiation creates a deepening and intimate link between the disciple and the Master of the lineage.
> – Rev. Kûban Jakkôin

Mikao Usui had performed these kinds of intense ascetic practices on Mt. Kurama and therefore was able to perform the mind-to-mind initiations. Let me emphasize this again: this kind of initiation can only be performed by a practitioner who has had a very direct experience of the True Self. Another word for initiation in Japan is *kaji* 加持 which translates as empowerment, blessing, grace or Buddha's power transferred to sentient beings. The kanji of *ka* can mean "to put on" while the kanji of *ji* means "holding." So we could say that *kaji* stands for "putting on the power of Buddha and holding it." The famous Shingon priest Ryuko Oda explains kaji as, "The transference of the Buddha's power or grace that inspires a sacred peace of mind and a strengthening of the life force." This is similar to what Mikao Usui was trying to point out as well. However, today's modern teachings seem so far removed from this older point of view.

We can only work with the grace of Buddha if we have seen our own Buddha nature or True Self, within ourselves. I cannot give you a cup of tea if I do not have one. This Buddha in *kaji* is Dainichi Nyorai, and Dainichi Nyorai is interlinked with Dai

Kômyô. From an esoteric Japanese perspective we could even say that if we have embodied the precepts as taught in the system of Reiki, we have embodied Dainichi Nyorai.

The explanation given for Dainichi Nyorai's participation in the world is that his grace (kaji) works to aid the practitioner to participate here and now in Dainichi Nyorai himself.
– David Edward Shaner, *The Bodymind Experience in Japanese Buddhism*

What is very interesting is that when I received a *kaji* from a Shugendo priest he focused on the same points as the Reiju I had learned within Mikao Usui's teachings. The *kaji* ritual itself had some differences, but I could see a clear similarity in it. Hiroshi Doi stated that he had seen about four slightly different Reiju rituals from traditional teachers in Mikao Usui's lineage. It is also very normal for differences to occur within *kaji* depending on the lineage, tradition, and teacher.

Mikkyo most often employs the four points of heart, forehead, throat, and crown of the head (in their traditional order), but many variations occur.
– Taiko Yamasaki, *Shingon Japanese Esoteric Buddhism*

Some other traditional points of focus within Mikkyo are the forehead, right shoulder, left shoulder, heart, and throat. These points also focus on similar points which Mikao Usui used in his hand-on healing sessions:

zento bu: forehead
sokuto bu: both sides of the head/temples
koutou bu: back of the head and forehead
enzui bu: neck (throat)
toucho bu: crown

This is one of the reasons why in Mikao Usui's time there was no difference between his Reiju and his hands-on healing sessions. They were both one and the same. However, this began to change when he started to teach students who were more interested in hands-on healing than rediscovering their True Self, like Chujiro Hayashi.

These points of focus often represent certain aspects, for example, the five senses, certain Buddhas, etc. Some of these five traditional esoteric aspects within *kaji* also link to the precepts. They are: ignorance and delusion, anger and hatred, pride and greed, desire and lust, and jealousy and fear. In this way, Reiju helps us to embody the precepts.

> That is to say, ideas of original enlightenment were not only transmitted through these initiation rites but embodied in their structure, iconography, and ritual gestures.
> – Jacqueline Stone, *Original Enlightenment and the Transformation of Medieval Japanese Buddhism*

However, what is most important within *kaji*, *kanjo*, and Reiju is not the physical ritual itself but the state of mind of the performer. If the state of mind of the performer is not in the right place then the whole ritual becomes just a mechanical procedure. Reiju, like *kaji* and *kanjo*, needs to be performed as much as possible from our True Self. This is why Mikao Usui taught the Dai Kômyô only to serious students when they were ready.

> With the practice of kaji what is most necessary to develop is peace of mind and purity, not just the ability to demonstrate "powers".
> – Ryuko Oda, *Kaji: Empowerment and Healing in Esoteric Buddhism*

The kind of Reiju, *kaji* or *kanjo* performed from this state of mind is not just an initiation but a healing as well. They are one and the same. This is because, as discussed numerous times within this book, real healing takes place in our mind. However, this began to change when Chujiro Hayashi focused his teachings more and more on the physical aspect of healing, away from the mind.

> Spiritual healing, kaji, in Esoteric Buddhism is not a medical practice. Its principle or purpose is to provide a sacred peace of mind.
> – Ryuko Oda, *Kaji: Empowerment and Healing in Esoteric Buddhism*

We can now slowly start to see that Mikao Usui borrowed his Reiju from traditional esoteric Japanese spiritual practices. In fact I believe that Mikao Usui was trying to make these esoteric teachings more available by simplifying them so that we all could rediscover our True Self. By delving deeper into practices like Shugendo, Shingon, Tendai, and Mikkyo, we can start to see from where Mikao Usui took his ideas and practices. This is one of the reasons I am studying with traditional Japanese priests: to get a clearer picture of what Mikao Usui was practicing himself and on what kind of teachings and philosophies he based his own teachings. There is much more to learn about Reiju and these kinds of connections, but those teachings are only for my students, in particular those who have been doing their training with me for a long period of time. Some things we cannot learn from a book.

Chapter 18

How to Give and Receive a Reiju

Within the kanji of the word Reiju we will find clues on how to receive and perform a spiritual blessing.

霊授 Reiju

How to give – 霊 Rei
The basic meaning of 霊 Rei is spiritual, but the deeper meaning is a shaman praying for rain, and the rains falls down. Within Japanese spiritual teachings the image of falling rain is often used to indicate certain aspects of the teachings. The first aspect is that the rain that is falling is of one flavor, one taste. This indicates that the essence of the universe is of one flavor, non-dual in nature. The second aspect is that when the rain falls it doesn't make any judgment about what a tree, a shrub, a flower, a field, a forest, needs; it just rains and they all take from it whatever they need at that time. Just let it rain and the client/student takes from the rain whatever he/she needs. This is the secret of how to give a Reiju: no need to judge, no need to label, just be open and let it rain. Reiju therefore is given from a state of mind of the precepts and the Dai Kômyô, from our True Self.

> We should work like the rain. The rain just falls. It doesn't ask, "Am I making a nice sound down below?" Or, "Will the plants be glad to see me? Will they be grateful?" The rain just falls, one raindrop after another. Millions and billions of raindrops only falling. This is the open secret of Zen.
> – Jakusho Kwong, *No Beginning, No End: The Intimate Heart of Zen*

If we do not come from this state of mind, we are not really performing a spiritual blessing or offering; we are just performing a ritual with no spirit in it at all. In Japan this kind of ritual is called an "empty ritual" because it is devoid of spirit, devoid of our True Self.

How to receive – 授 Ju
Ju 授 means: receive, hand down, give, impart, instruct, grant, offer, invest with, bless.

> This word, ju, is very good. "To cut," "to open," "to empty," and "to receive" are all expressed by ju.
> – Jakusho Kwong, *No Beginning, No End: The Intimate Heart of Zen*

Within the kanji of Ju lies the secret of how to receive. To really receive we need to be empty and open. I like to translate Ju as cut, because it is only after we cut that we are able to receive; the question is, what do we need to cut? We need to cut away all our attachments, all our preconceived ideas, or in other words we need to cut away our ego, the "I." When the "I" is out of the way we are completely empty and open and thus a perfect vessel to receive. We cannot receive anything if we are full of stuff, full of preconceived ideas about what we need to experience. Maybe we need to see colors, or feel energy, or get hot hands…all of these get in the way of really receiving. This means that by practicing all the meditation practices for ourselves we become empty vessels so that we can truly receive.

> When you receive something, you have to let go of everything, even yourself, the one who is receiving. Past, present – yes! even present! – and future, everything must go. Then we have true receiving.
> – Jakusho Kwong, *No Beginning, No End: The Intimate Heart of Zen*

These secret meanings hidden within the kanji of Reiju are therefore very important to understand and to embody. When we have the direct experience of Rei and Ju, then as a teacher we can just let it rain and as a receiver we can be utterly empty and open. Now we have a real spiritual blessing: Reiju.

Of course this concept is exactly the same during hands-on healing. If we are full of preconceived ideas, the "I" is in the way so we cannot receive. And if we do hands-on healing on others and we keep making judgments and labeling things, then we are not just letting it rain. I love how Mikao Usui used these kinds of words, like Reiki and Reiju, to indicate what he was trying to teach.

Chapter 19

What Is Real Giving and Receiving?

We often use the word "giving" when we talk about a Reiju or a hands-on healing session. But what is real giving? What is giving in accordance with the precepts? Giving in accordance with the precepts means that we give without anger and worry, from a place of being true to our way and our being, and in a state of mind of compassion.

Most of the time we do not give from this place: we have given with strings attached, and we expect something back. After we have given a Reiju, we want to hear how wonderful it was and what kind of amazing experiences our students had. And if they do not give this kind of feedback we either get worried that the Reiju didn't work or we get angry. Again this is the same for hands-on healing sessions and when we are teaching.

This is also why many of us do not like investigating questions from our students: we get worried or fearful that they do not trust the teachings, or maybe that they realize we do not know completely what we are teaching. Compassion is the key word within the precepts that will help us understand real spiritual giving. When we give from a state of mind of real compassion, we are giving without any strings attached. This means there is no need at all for anything to come back after we have given something: no "thank you," no explanations of what we saw or felt, nothing at all. Of course if it happens, that is fine, but if it doesn't happen then that is fine too. This is real giving. This kind of giving is compassionate giving because the "I" or ego is not involved.

How can we be compassionate if our ego is still part of giving? It is impossible. So even if we don't have this direct experience of letting go of the "I," we can at least understand it intellectually which is the first step. If we do not even understand this intellectually, then it is better if we do not give a Reiju, hands-on healing, or a teaching. When we let go of the "I" there is also no "mine" and when there is no "mine," there is also no "you." Thus in reality there is no "me" and nothing of mine to give and there is no "you" to receive. That is giving from the state of mind of real compassion and understanding the inner heart of the precepts.

> We say that the giver, receiver, and the gift itself are empty and peaceful. This is our standard for dana paramita [perfection of giving]: the giver is empty of self, the receiver is empty of self, and the thing given is empty of self. Simply selfless. Without this wisdom, giving is an ego trip. How can we cross over to a life where benefiting others is more important than our own self-interests? Unsurpassable giving is realizing that there is no one who possesses and that there is nothing to possess. When we realize this, giving and receiving is done without any thought of loss or gain.
> – Roshi Wendy Egyoku Nakao, Dharma Talk – "The Practice of Unsurpassable Giving"

The word "giving" is a tricky one. Imagine we have something in our hand. Now imagine that we give it to someone. Is your hand still holding it or is your hand empty? Our hand is empty. When we cling to giving from the viewpoint of the "I" and the ego, and we give something, then we feel we have also lost something. This is why a lot of practitioners or teachers feel tired after hands-on healing sessions, a Reiju, or teaching a class. This is because they feel they have given something and now they are empty. But if we come from the state of mind of the precepts, especially real compassion, and we realize that the giver, the gift, and the receiver are empty, then we can keep on doing hands-on healing, performing Reiju, or teaching. This kind of giving never depletes itself.

> In reflecting on dana paramita [perfection of giving], however, I am reminded that it requires "three kinds of purity." That is, according to Buddhism, true giving involves the awareness that there is no giver, no gift, and no receiver. Attachments of any kind – whether it be to self as the benefactor, the value of the gift, or the acknowledgment by the receiver – nullify the pure act of giving.
> – Taitetsu Unno, *Shin Buddhism: Bits of Rubble Turn into Gold*

We say, "I will give a Reiju and you will receive one." We have looked at different ideas of real giving, but what does real receiving mean? The word "receive" comes from the French word *receivre* which comes from the Latin word *recipere*, to take back. What are we taking back? When we receive a Reiju we are taking back our own power, our own great bright light. When we take back our own power, we start to stand in our own great bright light again, our True Self. Often we give away the power to a teacher or to someone else, and therefore we lose our own inner strength. But when we receive a real Reiju we take that power back, we take back what has always been there. This is real receiving. And don't forget, this is of course also related to hands-on healing!

Chapter 20

Spiritual Rain

Letting it rain is such an important teaching. Remember, Mikao Usui utilized the word Reiki. The Rei of Reiju is the same Rei as in Reiki. The kanji of Reiki is yet another pointer Mikao Usui put into his teachings. It is pointing towards how we need to perform a Reiju or a hands-on healing session. He put it there as a teaching: it is not merely the name of his teaching, but also another signpost. Thus we have to look at what the word Reiki as a signpost is pointing to and telling us.

The pre-1940s version of the kanji of Rei 靈 shows three little bowls or cups in a row. These bowls are often thought to represent the qualities of the trinity. This might be the trinity of the father, mother, and child; Earth, Heaven, and Oneness; or, if we look at the esoteric Japanese teachings, the three aspects of Buddha. Here again we can see a link between the word Reiki and the Okuden Reiki Level II mantras and their qualities. Another image within the kanji of Rei is that of a sorcerer praying for rain. Yes, we looked at this already in the previous chapter, but it is such an important element that I am going to repeat these teachings hidden within Rei.

Rain feeds our planet. Our world as we know it cannot exist without rain. In the kanji of Rei this nutritious, life-affirming rain falls down into the three bowls. This can be seen as the trinity being gifted with its fundamental nutritive needs. The practitioner/teacher (sorcerer) is connecting to the energy (rain), this energy pours down, and the client/student absorbs this energy for his or her fundamental needs. These needs, from a Japanese Reiki perspective, are the balancing elements within humanity of Earth, Heaven, and Oneness (the three bowls).

Imagine now a garden which has a couple of tall trees, beds

of colorful summer flowers, some shrubs, and a lovely lush, green stretch of grass. It begins to rain. At first big drops splatter on the leaves, the grass, the flower petals. And then it pours. Rain has only one flavor. It is rain. And rain does not make any distinction between the trees, the flowers, the shrubs, and the grass. There is no judgment in the rain. The rain does not think, "Well, look at that tall tree, I will rain a bit more on it and just a couple of drops on that little blade of grass." It is just rain. The tall tree, the flower, the shrub, and the blade of grass accept the rain according to their needs and ability to do so – not because the rain tells them what they can have and how they can have it. This is a very healthy and natural situation.

When we perform a treatment or *reiju*/initiation/attunement we need to act in this same way. The practitioner or teacher needs to "pray" for rain: praying in this sense is setting your intent, with the rain being the energy. The energy that we connect to as practitioners and teachers is only of one flavor, just like the rain. How can universal energy, which is non-dual in nature, have more flavors? As soon as we say, "This is a different kind of energy than that," then we are not talking about non-duality at all – thus also not about universal energy.

> *Though raindrops are many, they are of the same water*
> *Though rays of light are not one, they are of the same body*
> *The form and mind of that One are immeasurable*
> *The ultimate reality is vast and boundless*
> – Yoshito S. Hakeda, *Kukai: Major Works*

After we have set our intent and the energy starts to fall down we must make no judgments at all, just like the rain. The client/student will absorb the energy according to his or her needs and ability to do so, just like the tall trees, shrubs, flowers, and grass – not because the practitioner/teacher says so. As soon as a judgment is made about the client or student about the "amount" of Reiki they need, the practitioner/teacher is not coming from a place of love and compassion, and has stepped out of the healthy and natural flow. The process will therefore have a very different effect. One possible judgment that might be made during a treatment would be deciding that one particular spot needs more energy than another. Who are we to judge? Isn't it the client/student who decides what is needed? Thus we can see that the teachings within the word Reiki are pointing towards letting go of the "I," the ego, and therefore it is all about our True Self.

> When there is nothing in your mind, your ch'i is in harmony and tranquil. When your ch'i is in harmony and tranquil, it will be active and flowing, but it has no fixed form; and without using strength, it will naturally be strong.
> – Issai Chonzanshi, *The Demon's Sermon on the Martial Arts*, translated by William Scott Wilson

We have now discussed Rei; however, this rain is also pointed out in the kanji of Ki. Within the kanji of Ki, we see the word vapor, steam, or mist. The human body is made up of around 60% water. This is who we are physically. To create steam out of water we need fire or, in other words, heat. This fire will boil the water, which in turn creates steam. We also know that if we want to boil a pot of water, the fire needs to heat the pot from below – not the other way around. From this example we can see that the fire needs to come from our *hara*, our energetic center just below our navel, rather than from either our heaven – head – or heart centers.

At an energetic level our dense water energy, which is more like frozen water due to our anger, worries, fears, and useless attachments, begins to melt. It becomes subtler and subtler, turning into steam, and gradually it starts to rise. When it has risen as far as it can go, it transforms itself into rain. This rain then falls back from our crown down into our *hara*, creating a continuous movement between the earth and heavenly energy.

This cycle of transforming water into steam and letting the steam rain down to nurture us is a replica of what we see in nature. The water on earth is heated up by the sun, which makes it rise as mist, the mist creates clouds, which creates rain, which then falls back down onto the earth to nurture it, allowing everything to bloom. When this happens we have become intimate with nature because we are a microcosm within the macrocosm. The universe is us and we are the universe, no separation. In many traditions this rain is called inner happiness or inner bliss.

The inner fire within the *hara* is facilitated by prolonged practices like *joshin kokyu hō* and chanting the mantra *choku rei*. If we look very closely at each individual sounds of the mantras *choku rei, sei heki, hon sha ze sho nen,* and Dai Kômyô, we can start to see clearly fire and water in them as well. As I said before, there are many hidden messages and teachings within each tool. Our task as practitioners and teachers is to rediscover these meanings and have a direct experience of them so that we can become better practitioners and teachers.

Chapter 21

The Umbrella

In essence, spiritual rain falls down all the time, but we seem to hold up an umbrella all the time as well. This means that we prevent ourselves from being nurtured by this spiritual rain. The umbrella represents our attachments, worries, fear, insecurities and so on. In fact we can say that the umbrella is the same as the lampshades. How do we let go of the umbrella and let the spiritual rain bless us all the time? The first steps in this process are taught within Shoden Reiki Level I: the precepts and the meditation practice of *joshin kokyu hō*. Without this foundation it is difficult to awaken the flow of energy that triggers this inner happiness. By practicing this meditation daily, the seat of our original energy – our *hara* – is stirred.

Practicing the methods taught within Okuden Level II helps us to loosen our grip on the umbrella a bit more. The initial Okuden practice of meditating on the first symbol and/or mantra stimulates the earth connection through the *hara* even further. After establishing a good connection with the earth energy you move on to work with the next symbol and/or mantra which symbolizes heavenly energy, associated with your head. After both the heaven and earth energy are in perfect harmony, something begins to shift within your inner energetic system. This shift is paired with feeling heat within the *hara*. When our heaven and earth energy is in harmony, the heat from the *hara* rises all the way to the head. This in turn melts the heavenly energy in our head, which in turn drips down through our central channel and into our heart.

The inner heat rising is called Ri Goma in Japan and is a fundamental practice in all Japanese spiritual teachings. When this starts to happen, it is time to begin to meditate with the third

Okuden symbol and/or mantra: related to your heart/mind. The energy that drips down from your head into the heart continues dripping down into the *hara*. This blossoming of the three energy centers stimulates an inner blossoming of happiness. The more we work with this, the more inner happiness blossoms and spreads through the entire body. Initially, you might begin to feel a gentle inner heat and a tingling sensation flowing through you. This is enhanced by meditating on the Shinpiden Level III symbol and/or mantra, bringing the blossoming to fruition. There is now a continual flow of energy from the *hara* to your head and back down again. This flow of energy is the rain pointed out by Mikao Usui.

> The training according to the Natural Law of this whole world develops human spirituality. When you are convinced of this Truth, your committed training actualizes the unification with the Universe. The word you speak and the action you take becomes One with the Universe and they effortlessly work as the absolute limitlessness. This is in other words, the true nature of the human.
> – 会員のみに配布する霊気療法のしおり– Usui Reiki Ryôhô Gakkai, "Leaflet of Reiki Ryôhô – Members Only"

This kind of rain is a Reiju, a spiritual blessing, and is called Muso-Sanmitsu Kaji (a formless blessing from the three mysteries of the universe). It is our state of mind of inner bliss – a sense of aliveness coming deep from within ourselves. Or in other words we have laid bare the great bright light of our True Self, and this light creates the heat and energy/tingling throughout our whole being.

Here is a simple metaphor to help us to understand this concept of real aliveness. Imagine a wire, stripped of its plastic coating but not connected to the power supply. Nothing happens when we touch it as there is no energy running through it. This is a dead wire. Yet, when we insert the wire into the outlet and then touch it, we feel the energy of the electricity. This is known as a live wire.

So, to be alive we need to be like the wire, feeling the energy moving through us all the time. When we feel this movement of energy creating inner happiness and joy, it makes us want to announce to the world: I am alive! But here is the catch: If our internal wires are old and not often used and we suddenly plug ourselves into this unlimited power source called the universe, what will happen to the wires?

So here is the next metaphor: Imagine an old wire running from the power point to a lamp. Within the lamp is a 40-watt light bulb. Now we switch on the light and all is fine, no problem at all. But let's change the 40-watt light bulb to a 100-watt bulb and then switch on the light. What will happen to the old wires? They will burn as they cannot handle the amount of energy. This is a really important element within these teachings. For most of us, we cannot suddenly switch on the great bright light of our True Self, because our mind, body, and energy will not be able to handle it. This is why the system of Reiki is divided into three distinct levels; each level will help our mind, body, and energy to become stronger and more stable so that one day when we finally let go of the umbrella or uncover the last lampshade of our True Self, we will be fine.

The closer we come to rediscovering our True Self, the more the rain will fall, and we will slowly start to become Reiju. Eventually we throw the umbrella away so it can rain 24 hours a day. This is the real Reiju Mikao Usui was pointing out: a continuous flow of spiritual blessings. This is also the Reiju Mikao Usui himself experienced during his 21-day meditation practice on Mt. Kurama. All of this brings us to Part V of this book, called "Practice," because it is only through understanding and experiencing the practices that we throw away the umbrella for good.

Part V

Practice

Chapter 22

How Do We Learn?

Most of us know that people learn in many different styles, such as kinesthetic, visual, auditory, and intellectual. Mikao Usui also knew this and adjusted his teachings accordingly. Let's look at each one of these and see how it relates to his teachings. Remember that one is not better than the other, just a different way. For example, if you want to enter a room that is filled with beautiful energy, does it matter if you enter through the visual door, the auditory door, the intellectual door, or the kinesthetic door? Of course not, as long as you are able to enter the room.

Mikao Usui's intellectual teaching tools are the precepts; we need to intellectually understand them before we can also start to embody them with our whole being. If we do not even understand intellectually what it means to be kind or compassionate, then it will be very difficult to embody this. Some of the concepts that Mikao Usui would have transmitted orally would have also fallen under this heading. We often first listen to or read some teachings, but that is not enough. We then need to contemplate them to see if they make sense. Many teachers write or say things and we take them for granted. I ask that you don't take anything in this book for granted either; investigate, contemplate, and see if it all makes sense.

Even contemplation is not enough, because we also need to gain the direct experience of it. For example I might say Choku Rei is connected to earth energy; you can just take that for granted, but that is not very wise. You can contemplate what I say and ask yourself if it makes sense. But in the end you need to meditate with the Choku Rei yourself for months and see what your direct experience is. Then and only then can you know if what I have said is true or not. If we do not experience these things directly, then we will never truly know them.

The visual aspects in Usui's teachings are the Reiki symbols. Traditionally they were there to meditate upon as a visual aid and were not used externally. They were there to help you to become more mindful and to help you remember your True Self. The student would sit in meditation and draw the symbol in his mind again, again, and again, so that he would not be distracted by the past, present, and future. By practicing this over and over one would ultimately become the symbol. Another visual aspect of Usui's teachings can be seen in the meditation practices, like *joshin kokyu hō*. During this meditation the student visualizes bringing bright energy into the *hara* and then expanding it through his whole being.

Why would visualizing yourself as a symbol or as a bright light be helpful? It would help you to let go of the "I," replacing it with a symbol or a bright light. Practicing this every day helps soften the grip on the "I," which in turn helps us to rediscover our own pure potential, our True Self. It is only after we let go of the "I" that we can embody the precepts. It is the "I" who is getting angry; it is the "I" who is getting worried and fearful. It is the "I" who is getting in the way of being compassionate to ourselves and others.

> Concentrating on a sound or object encourages attention, a stepping stone to satori, and learning to concentrate is vital for experiencing satori.
> – H. E. Davey, *The Teachings of Tempu: Practical Meditation for Daily Life*

This letting go of the "I" was also the aim of the auditory teachings of Mikao Usui. The auditory elements within his teachings are the mantras that we have discussed in detail in some of the previous chapters. Chanting a mantra is extremely beneficial and used in all major spiritual traditions inside and outside Japan. When we chant the mantra we need to focus all our intention on the way we chant it. Chanting while daydreaming about the past, present, or future will take us nowhere. The mantra will only show its inner heart when we repeat the mantra with all our focused intention again and again for many weeks, months, or years. For many people, chanting will be more physical than working with a visual aid. For this reason, chanting is an extremely important tool, especially for beginners, who often want to feel something. In the beginning, not feeling anything during practice might be discouraging; however, over time we start to have the direct insight that our practice is not about feeling anything but about becoming a more compassionate person.

> *A mantra is supranational.*
> *It eliminates ignorance when meditated upon and recited.*
> *A single word contains a thousand truths.*
> *One can realize Suchness here and now.*
> *Walk on and on until quiescence is reached.*
> *Go on and on until the primordial Source is penetrated.*
> – Yoshito S. Hakeda, *Kukai: Major Works*

Kinesthetic learning is therefore also an important element within Mikao Usui's teachings, especially for beginners: physically placing the hands on or slightly off the body. If you asked a beginner to just sit together with his client without any physical movement or touch, he would find that very difficult. However, a dedicated practitioner within Mikao Usui's teachings would have no issue with this. This is also why in modern practices the system of Reiki has become more and more tactile; not many practitioners take the time to delve deeper into the heart of the teachings, into the heart/mind connection.

It is good to remember that hands-on healing is just a tool. When we place our hands on a client's knee, where is the client's mind going? Your client's mind is going to the knee because she feels a hand there. So where is her energy going? It goes also to the knee, as energy follows the mind. Where is your own mind and energy going when you place your hand on your heart center, for example? Investigate this and see what happens. However, our mind is always so busy and gets quickly distracted, thus we have to keep focusing on the hand on our body. When we do this over and over, our mind can start to stay focused for longer periods of time. And after many years of practice we can even let go of placing the hands on our body. You might be lying down and set your intent that you want to heal yourself and that you receive whatever you need and suddenly you feel all this energy flowing through your whole being. Now you have "become" the hand positions.

Some students need a combination of these different ways of learning, while others are happy to stick with one specific way. This all depends on who we are and what our inclinations are. The most important thing to remember is not the methods themselves, but that through these methods we learn how to become more mindful and that over time we start to rediscover our True Self. A good teacher would be able to guide the student towards his True Self with these kinds of teachings and practices.

All the above practices focus on a specific tool: a mantra, a visualization, a breathing method, a physical posture, a precept, or a ritual. These kinds of practices are called practices with form (Jp. *uso*) because they focus on a specific method. But because we cannot always practice with form, they are really just signposts until we reach a state in which we can "practice" without form (Jp. *muso*). When we reach a state of *muso* we are resting our mind in the great bright light, our True Self. Now life becomes meditation and meditation becomes life. At this stage there is nothing to practice; we just *Be* Reiki.

Just as the highest initiation has no set format, the ultimate

Mikkyo practice is the "formless," spontaneous activity of wisdom expressed not in ritual but in the complexity of day-to-day life.
– Taiko Yamasaki, *Shingon Japanese Esoteric Buddhism*

However, we need to be very careful about throwing away the form practices too quickly. Even if we can be in the no-form practice, we might have to use some form practices as well, depending on the day or if we practice with a client or student who still needs the form practices. For example, if we reach a state of no-form and we get a client for hands-on healing who is not in the right state of mind for a no-form session, we still need to use the form practice of the physical hand positions. From this perspective we need to reach a state in which the form and no-form practice are in harmony with each other.

If practitioners discard their various practices and seek to dwell only in that without form they will not succeed. On the other hand, neither will they succeed if they cling to their practice, seeking to dwell in that which has form.
– Commentary on the Dainichi-kyo

Chapter 23

Different Tools, Same Thing

In the previous chapter we looked at the different ways of learning and how Mikao Usui put these in his teachings. But that is not all. He was very clever; the different ways were not really different: they did the same thing. Let's explore this a bit deeper because if we start to understand this, we can take Mikao Usui's teachings to a whole different level.

Let's look at *hatsurei hō*, a fundamental meditation practice taught within Okuden Level II. *Hatsurei hō* has been translated in many ways, but the heart of it is about remembering our True Self. This meditation practice consists of three different elements:

Kenyoku Hō

1. *Gassho* – to center the mind and set intent while standing or sitting. Take a few deep breaths into the *hara*.
2. Place your right hand on the left shoulder. Breathe in, and on the out-breath, sweep diagonally down from the left shoulder to right hip.
3. On the in-breath, place your left hand on the right shoulder and, on the out-breath, sweep down diagonally from right shoulder to left hip.
4. Breathe in, returning your right hand to the left shoulder and, on the out-breath, sweep diagonally down from left shoulder to right hip.
5. With the left elbow against your side, and with your arm horizontal to the ground, place your right hand on the left forearm. Breathe in and, on the out-breath, sweep downward along the arm to the fingertips and out.
6. With the right elbow against your side and with your right arm horizontal to the ground, place your left hand on the

right forearm. Breathe in and – on the out-breath – sweep down along the arm to the fingertips and out.

7. Breathe in and, with the left elbow against your side and with your arm horizontal to the ground, place your right hand on the left forearm. On the out-breath, sweep down along the arm to the fingertips and out.

8. *Gassho* – to give thanks.

Joshin Kokyu Hō

1. Place your hands in your lap, palms facing upwards.

2. With each in-breath feel the energy coming in through the nose, move the energy and your mind down to the *hara*, expand the energy and your mind through your entire body.

3. On the out-breath, expand the energy and your mind out of the body, through your skin and continue to expand out into your surroundings.

4. Repeat steps 2 and 3 until finished. The exercise may take anywhere from 5 minutes to half an hour.

5. *Gassho* – to give thanks.

Seishin Toitsu

1. With your hands in the *gassho* position, focus on your *hara*. On the in-breath, begin to bring the energy into your hands. Feel the energy move along your arms, down though your body and into the *hara*. Make sure your mind stays focused on this movement.

2. On the out-breath, visualize energy moving from the *hara* back up through the body and then to the arms and out through the hands. Make sure your mind stays focused on the movement.

3. Repeat for as long as you wish.

4. *Gassho* – to give thanks.

If we look closely at the *hatsurei hō* we see a few very interesting things. *Kenyoku hō* is about grounding yourself in a simple yet effective way. This takes place as we sweep downwards, and also because when we sweep our body, we physically touch ourselves which in turn helps us to stay in our body and not drift off with the fairies. So we could say it is the beginning of learning how to ground oneself. To take this grounding and connecting to the earth even deeper, we do *joshin kokyu hō*. During *joshin kokyu hō* we breathe deep into the *hara*; this has the same effect as working with the mantra *choku rei*. Some of Mikao Usui's students had difficulty with the mantra *choku rei* so he taught them *joshin kokyu hō*: different method, same outcome. *Kokyu* is our in- and out-breath: *ko* is the exhalation and *kyu* is the inhalation. When we breathe properly, we breathe like a newborn baby, with our belly. In this way we become centered and grounded.

Seishin toitsu is about the heavenly energy being grounded in the *hara*, which harmonizes heaven and earth energy. One of the meanings of *toitsu* is harmony, therefore harmony is also the quality of *sei heki*. Another meaning of *toitsu* is focused. During this meditation practice we place our hands in *gassho*, which in turn will focus our mind on the more upper regions of our body, since the tips of the fingers are in line with the tip of our nose. This upper part of our body represents the heavenly energy (*sei heki*) while the breathing into the *hara* represents the earth energy (*choku rei* – focus). Mind and body become one as seen in the precepts: *Shinshin kaizen* – "Create harmony between your mind and body."

It is this place and this state of mind I come to when my spirit (Seishin) is gathered (Toitsu), when my mind (Seishin) is one (Toitsu). Gone are the myriad distractions and all that remains is myself, focused and attentive on the here and now. All is equal and in harmony and this transcends all.
– Erik Takase, *Kampsport*, 1999 Issue

We can now start to see that the different components of *hatsurei hō* look different than the mantras of *choku rei* and *sei heki*, but that in fact they do exactly the same thing! When we practice *hatsurei hō* in its complete form, we have the mantra *hon sha ze sho nen*. The meditation practice helps us to have a direct experience of I am Right Mind. To sum it all up, *hatsurei hō* is a kinesthetic and visual practice that does the same thing as working with the three auditory mantras taught within Okuden Level II. Plus we also see that *hatsurei hō* points towards the precepts. When our innate earth and heavenly energy are more in harmony, we get less angry and worried. When we unify them completely, we can experience Oneness, which in turn helps us with being compassionate.

The mantras are also interlinked with the precepts; they are again one and the same thing. Let's take a look at the quality of *sei heki*, which is harmony. When we are in harmony with the universe what will drop away? Fear and worry will drop away because we are now in harmony with all that is. If we say we have realized that we are one with the universe, and yet we still feel the need to protect ourselves, then our realization is only intellectual and not an embodiment. If we have embodied harmony, then we have also embodied the precept, "Do not worry."

When our mind is in complete harmony with the cosmic order...then we have nothing more to fear.
– Taisen Deshimaru, *Mushotoku Mind: The Heart of the Heart Sutra*

All the other elements within Mikao Usui's teachings are exactly the same, but to explain this is beyond the scope of this book, and it is also better to seek direct experiences. We cannot learn everything from a book; this is just the beginning, and to learn the deeper elements I invite you to take a class.

Chapter 24

Ready or Not Ready

Mikao Usui taught each student according to his or her spiritual progress, and this is also why there are different ideas, practices, and precepts within his teachings. Again one is not better than the other, just a different way. We need to find the way that suits each of us as an individual. This might also change over time. Perhaps at first you are only interested in hands-on healing, but over time you suddenly find that you want to go deeper and want to embody the teachings more. Maybe your current teacher can help you if she or he has gone that path her or himself. But if he or she hasn't because of his/her own readiness, you might need to find a different teacher who will help you to go deeper.

This is the best example I can give you about being ready. It is a story about a peach tree and peach season. If there is a peach tree and it is peach season are all the peaches ripe at the same time? No, it all depends where the peaches have been hanging: in the sun or shade, by themselves or in a cluster. We are like the peaches in the peach tree – some are more ripe than others. This of course is not bad or good, it is just the way it is. Now we can ask ourselves another question: How do you get the ripe peaches out of the tree? In fact the ripest peach will fall out all by itself; we can just sit with the tree and see the ripest peach fall out. But if there is no peach on the ground or we do not have the time to just be with the tree, what do we need to do?

We gently shake the tree and the ripest peach will fall out. For the not-so-ripe peach, we need to shake the tree much harder. And for the peach that is not ripe at all, we might need to get an external object, like some scissors, and cut it loose from the branch.

Our clients, our students and we ourselves are exactly the same. If we have a very ripe client, all we need to do is gently give them a nudge and healing starts to take place. This nudge could be just to ask our client to set their intent that they want to heal themselves and that they will receive whatever they need for the healing to take place, and that is all that is needed. Or if we have a student, all we might need to do is sit with our student and the reiju/initiation/attunement will take place. But of course most of the time this is not the case. This is why many practices and methods have become more elaborate, even using certain implements. This of course also depends heavily on the practitioner's or teacher's own readiness. If the practitioner or teacher is not a ripe peach and the client is not a ripe peach then you might need to use lots of implements, for example. But if the teacher is very ripe and the student is ripe then all you have to do is be with each other and healing or reiju/initiation/attunement can take place.

> Confucius said, "I am not going to go on with the fellow who does not respond by lifting up three corners when I have already lifted up one."
> – Issai Chonzanshi, The Demon's Sermon on the Martial Arts, translated by William Scott Wilson

How do we become ripe? Like the peach tree we need the rain and the light of the universe to get ripe. But by just sitting back and thinking that it will rain on us or the sun will shine on us, nothing is going to take place. We need to actively engage with the universe and therefore we need to actively practice the meditation techniques Mikao Usui implemented in his teachings. This is also why the rain and sun are emphasized again and again in Mikao Usui's teachings, the rain of Reiki and Reiju, and the great bright light of Dai Kômyô.

But having said this, even though there are different stages in our ripeness, one's True Self is always ready and always bright, no matter what. It is only due to our lampshades and umbrellas that we have these different kinds of readinesses.

Chapter 25

The System of Reiki Is Meditation

All the practices within the system of Reiki are meditation practices. If we have not built a good foundation, then we cannot work with the deeper teachings. Those deeper teachings will in fact become confusing and might even unbalance us more. This is why Mikao Usui taught different levels; each level is a building block for the next. The meditation practices taught within each of these levels are also building blocks.

But what is meditation? Many people get confused about what meditation really is.

The first misconception is that when we meditate we should not have any thoughts in our mind. But this of course is impossible, because if we have no thoughts we become like a zombie. Ask yourself, "How do I get up from my sitting practice if I have no thought to get up?" We will always have thoughts in our minds, but through practicing meditation techniques we can learn how not to cling to them. The key word here is cling; it is so easy to get caught up in thought patterns. We follow our thoughts when we cling to the past, to the future, and even to the present moment. When we follow our thoughts, getting tangled up like cling wrap, we suffer from anger, fears, worries and all sorts of attachments. If we experience thoughts coming up and we don't cling to them, then we are free; the thoughts will dissolve back to the place they came from, leaving no trace of anger, fear, worry or other attachments. Now this of course is not that easy, and therefore we work with meditation practices and techniques to support this.

Let me state it clearly: don't be afraid of wandering thoughts, and do not waste your energy subduing them, don't follow them, and don't try to get rid of them. As long as you do not continue wallowing in them, wandering thoughts will naturally depart themselves.

– Xunyun, in Sheng Yen, *Attaining the Way: A Guide to the Practice of Chan Buddhism*

As you can see, I call them meditation practices and techniques because this is where another misconception comes in, and that is that there is only one way to meditate: sitting down on a meditation pillow, as would a monk or a nun. Meditation is in fact not a physical position, but rather a state of mind, free from dualistic thinking. It is a direct experience of our True Self. Thus meditation is life, and life is meditation. The heart of meditation is resting our mind in the great bright light of Dai Kômyô, because when we rest our mind in this non-dual state we can walk, talk, drive a car and still be in meditation. But of course to have this direct experience of being free from our dualistic thinking is once again not that easy, therefore we use more meditation practices and techniques. These meditation practices and techniques have many different forms. They can be performed when sitting, moving, and sitting and moving.

At different times during our lives we might need to work with different forms, depending on how our practice is developing. If we only use a sitting meditation practice or technique we might find it very difficult to maintain the state of being free of dualistic thinking while we are walking. Therefore we need to use both so that we learn how to engage in the world while our mind rests in a non-dualistic state. Performing the *reiju*/initiation/attunement and/or hands-on healing from this meditative state is an excellent tool for learning how to move while we are still being mindful. This means that with lots of practice and perseverance one can learn to live life in a state of mind of meditation, free from clinging, free from attachments, and free from dualistic thinking. Thus no matter if we walk, talk, brush our teeth, shit, laugh, sit, or sleep, our mind is free, and this is the deepest form of meditation of all.

> Real meditation involves doing nothing and resting in complete naturalness.
> – H. E. Davey, *The Teachings of Tempu: Practical Meditation for Daily Life*

Therefore all the meditation practices within the system of Reiki – the precepts, breathing meditations, hands-on healing, symbols and mantras, and the *reiju*/initiation/attunement – are signposts to help us to "become" meditation, or in other words remember our True Self.

Chapter 26

Meditating on the Precepts

So how can we practice with the precepts? Many teachers say that all we need to do is just say the precepts three times a day and that is about it. But even if I say "I am happy" three times a day, that wouldn't necessarily make me a happy person. If it was that easy the world would be a different place by now with no more anger, worry, and fear, and filled with love and compassion. All we have to do is say "I am happy" a few times a day and hey presto the world is a better place. But we all know that is not the case. We need to honestly look at our practice and see if what we are being taught has the effect we are looking for.

> Memorizing a definition of the truth isn't personally seeing the truth. It is second-hand understanding. It's neither your experience nor your knowledge. Regardless how much material is remembered, and no matter how eloquently we speak about remembered information, we're devoted to a description of something that's not ours. Besides, the description is never the item itself. Clinging to our impression of particular descriptions or teachings, we're often unable to see the real thing when it's right before our eyes. Our eyes are conditioned by our memorization of, and convictions about, topics we've never seen for ourselves. This is prevalent enough as to be the rule.
> – H. E. Davey, *The Teachings of Tempu: Practical Meditation for Daily Life*

My favorite three practices with the precepts are repetition, pulling it apart, and throwing it in the air. All three of them are meditation practices. I would suggest that you take one precept at a time. For example, work with "Do not anger" for a month or so before you move on to the next precept. This way you get to really delve much deeper into the heart of the teachings and gaining a direct experience of "Do not anger."

For the repetition practice, sit in your favourite meditation position, take a few deep breaths, and start to repeat the precept "Do not anger" for maybe 10 minutes. When we repeat it again and again we have to stay focused on what we are repeating, thus it helps us not to get distracted by the past, present, and future. Afterwards just sit for a minute or so quietly; be mindful of whether or not you get distracted.

For the "pulling it apart" practice, sit in meditation and start to pull the precept "Do not anger" apart. Ask yourself questions like, "Who is it who gets angry? Who is this 'I' who gets angry? Can I find this 'I'? What happens when I get angry?" Do this for about 10 minutes. Investigate and keep pulling it apart till there is nothing to pull apart anymore. Afterwards just sit quietly and mindfully in that space.

> In Buddhism we use the words no or not to show that nothing has its own separate existence, everything is interconnected and produced by interdependent co-origination.
> – Dainin Katagiri, *Each Moment Is the Universe*

For the "throwing it in the air" practice, sit in meditation, take a few deep breaths and wait till your mind feels like a calm lake. Now throw the precept "Do not anger" into the air and let it fall into your lake-like state of mind. What kind of ripples can you see, feel, or experience? Don't intellectualize it, don't label it, just observe. Sit in this ripple effect for 10 minutes. If we feel we start to follow the ripples or we start to think about something else, take a few breaths again and return to the nature of mind which is like a lake. Ripples do not form if we throw something in a stormy sea. So for this meditation practice to be successful we first need to make our mind as calm as a lake.

These practices help us to look deeper at our anger, worry, and fear, and why we are not compassionate. Some might say that the word "not" within the precepts "Do not anger" and "Do not worry" will in fact bring up anger and worry. Like the concept of, "Do not think of a pink elephant" and you start to think of a pink elephant. They therefore replace these precepts with something else, like: I am kind, or I am free.

But it is in fact a good thing that we bring up our anger and worry, because when we bring it up we can do something about it. If we don't even know we have anger, worry, or fear within us, how can we start to do something about it; we are ignorant about our issues. Insight into our own issues is a must; it is wisdom, which we can utilize to be able to start to remember our True Self.

Normally we are like a rubber boat moving on the sea. Suddenly we hear *pfff* and we discover a little leak in our boat. We quickly patch it up with a patch and keep going. A day or a few weeks later we hear another *pfff*, and we discover yet another leak in our boat. Again we patch it up and just keep going, until one day our rubber boat has so many leaks and patches that it has become a very weak and unstable rubber boat. Wouldn't it make more sense to go straight to the root of why we get leaks in the first place instead of patching them up again and again?! By bringing up our own inner anger, worries, and fears we gain insights into why we have them. We go straight to the root instead of patching them up with saying "I am kind" while we still have not dealt with our anger.

Only by confronting suffering as it is and by becoming clearly aware of its origins, does it become possible to step beyond it.
– Ryuko Oda, *Kaji: Empowerment and Healing in Esoteric Buddhism*

Chapter 27

Hands-on Healing as Meditation

One of the reasons that Mikao Usui taught hands-on healing on ourselves is that it is a very physical kinesthetic practice. Some of Mikao Usui's later students appeared less interested in meditation practices like *joshin kokyu hō* or chanting mantras, as their world was opening up and being influenced by Western cultures. To be able to guide them he also started to introduce hands-on healing in his teachings. This hands-on healing practice evolved over time to become a more externalized practice, and today many of us have forgotten the inner/hidden (Jp. *ura*) meaning of hands-on healing for ourselves. What is the inner/hidden meaning of hands-on self-healing? What is the heart of it?

The first thing we need to ask ourselves is what is happening in our minds when we place our hands on ourselves. The mind is the most important element within hands-on healing. When I touch my body I am both the person who is touching and the person who is being touched. This sensation within our mind triggers a letting go of the "I." This happens because we find it difficult to realize that we are touching and being touched at the same time by our own body, so we let go. On the deepest level it helps trigger a state of non-duality or, in other words, we rediscover our True Self. However, this can only happen when we stay mindful during hands-on healing on ourselves, and do not fall asleep during it.

Ichiwaka Hiroshi, a Japanese contemporary philosopher, states it very beautifully in his book *Seishin Toshite no Shintai* [The Body as the Spirit]: "Although I am touching myself who is [also] being touched, this doubling of sensations is further internalized to enable me to discover myself who takes note of touching, which invites me to a purification of the thought that 'I am touching.'"

The more we purify the notion of "I am touching," the more we can let go of the "I." Yet this can only start to happen when we are mindful during the process of hands-on healing. This will not take place when we perform hands-on healing on ourselves while watching TV or when our mind is all over the place. Consequently, it is only if we are mindful during the process that hands-on healing on ourselves becomes meditation. Meditation is when our mind is not being distracted by the past, future, or even by the present. In this way we are also creating a very intimate relationship with ourselves, as intimacy only happens when there is a mutual agreement between two elements, which means we feel no difference between what is being touched and the toucher. For example, if I touch a tree and I feel there is a big difference between the tree and me, intimacy will not take place. However, when I let go of the notion of "I am touching the tree," the "I" and the "tree," then we can become intimate, and finally reach a state of non-duality. The more we let go of the "I," the more we can reach into this state of non-duality. The kind of intimacy we are discussing here we can find back in the precept chapter where I explained the kanji of kindness. We are being kind to ourselves, meaning we are becoming intimate with our True Self.

Suzuki-roshi taught that real intimacy means through and through; a way of living our daily lives, rooted in the practice of Zen, so that everything is included in what we do, and yet we leave no trace. When we live with this kind of intimacy, we are always expressing our true self, the wholeness of our original nature, which has neither beginning nor end.
– Jakusho Kwong, *No Beginning, No End: The Intimate Heart of Zen*

All of Mikao Usui's teachings, including hands-on healing, point in the same direction, letting go of the "I." Because it is only when we let go of the "I" that we rediscover our True Self. We might think that hands-on healing was developed to alleviate our physical pain, but that is really only the outer meaning of hands-on healing. The inner/hidden meaning is letting go of the "I." Because when we let go of the "I," then there is no "I" who is worried about the pain and discomfort.

This letting go of the "I" is also seen within *gassho* (prayer position); in fact gassho is a kind of hands-on healing on ourselves. Gassho is placing our hands together in a praying position. This position is about the left hand touching the right hand and the right hand touching the left hand – the toucher being touched. Which further helps us to let go of the notion of "I," bringing us deeper into a state of mind of non-duality.

> In many religions, the reason that one closes his eyes, and joins his hands together when he prays is because he attempts to reach by way of his activity a certain pure state that is without fissure between activity and passivity, between interiority and exteriority, and between subject and object.
> – Ichiwaka Hiroshi, *Seishin Toshite no Shintai* [The Body as the Spirit]

It is only when we let go of the notion of subject and object, toucher and being touched, that we can rediscover our True Self. This is also the inner heart of hands-on healing on others, but we can only really start to see this if we have had a direct experience of this during hands-on healing on ourselves. When we perform hands-on healing on others we might say, "I am doing Reiki and I am touching my client." But if you are touching your client, then the client is also touching you. The toucher becomes the one who is being touched, and the person who is being touched will also become the toucher. Normally we only see things from a dualistic perspective, so we either touch or we are being touched. Our confused mind finds it very difficult to realize that we are both touching and being touched at the same time when we are doing hands-on healing on others. This understanding of being the toucher and being touched is the direct experience of harmony, unity of two dualistic elements.

You are now currently holding either a book or an electronic device to read this book. You might say, "I am touching my book," or, "I am touching my kindle." But take a moment to reflect on this because the book or kindle is also touching you. When we start to see hands-on healing on others from this perspective, we also start to see something else happening. We start to see and feel that our hands are just the beginning. If the "I" falls away, then our "client, "you," will also fall away. This means that we are now being intimate, heart to heart, from True Self to True Self. Of course this is not that easy, and this is why Mikao Usui taught his students according to their spiritual progress and understanding. A beginner might not have these kinds of experiences. They first need to work on creating a solid foundation within themselves. But a practitioner or teacher who delves deep into his/her True Self will understand these kinds of teachings and experiences. Now hands-on healing becomes a meditation practice. Now we can just Be with our client, even if we move our hands.

> In reality, hand positions have nothing whatsoever to do with the deeper process of healing. Hands are a very superficial way for humans to connect to energy when we are first learning. The true power of energy, however, lies in the ability to completely let go of our reliance on our hands and allow the energy to flow throughout our entire body. More than that, we must learn to allow the energy to flow even deeper – beyond our physical bodies and into our minds and spirits.
> – Kathleen Prasad, *Reiki for Dogs*

If we do not see hands-on healing as a meditation we might start to believe that we can do hands-on healing while we watch TV or talk. But if this was the case why did Mikao Usui put practices like *hatsurei hō* and *joshin kokyu hō* into his system?

> Hatsurei Ho has been handed down starting with Usui Sensei as a practice of self-purification and spiritual growth leading to enlightenment.
> – Hiroshi Doi, *A Modern Reiki Method for Healing*

Joshin kokyu hō means "breathing technique to purify your mind." *Kokyu* also means "movement of your ki" and "focused power." Mikao Usui is pointing towards the mind and focus. Practicing these meditations creates a focused mind by requiring concentration and intention. If our mind is all over the place while we are talking and watching TV then we have no power in our ki, as the mind is very distracted and unfocused. Another thing to consider is that when we do talk or watch TV during treatments, it is often about things which are based on worries and fear, or just idle gossip; this in turn takes us away from being in the state of mind of the precepts.

> When mind moves, ki moves.
> – Yuasa Yasuo, *The Body, Self-Cultivation, and Ki-Energy*

Imagine that during treatment you are thinking of going afterwards to your favorite coffee shop to get a chai latte and a chocolate brownie. Ask yourself: Where is my mind? Your mind is at the coffee shop in the future. Thus where is your energy? Also in the coffee shop and in the future, which means you are not focused and with your client. To really be with your client you need to be focused! This is called being mindful. One of the teachings of the inner heart of the system of Reiki is mindfulness.

Mind and ch'i are fundamentally of one essence. If you were to speak of separating them, they would be like fire and firewood.
– Issai Chonzanshi, *The Demon's Sermon on the Martial Arts*, translated by William Scott Wilson

In a very direct way we can say that our energy follows the mind. To gain a clear, focused, open, and expanded energy we need to work with the mind. It is only the really advanced practitioner who is in the real state of mind of non-duality who can talk and watch TV while still being focused. Why? Because this kind of practitioner is not judging things as good or bad, positive or negative, here or there, thus she will be not swayed by all the emotions, distractions, and attachments.

Hands-on healing needs to be a form of meditation, where we are mindful and focused. Performing hands-on healing on others should come from our own personal practice. The more lampshades we take away from our own innate great bright light, the brighter our light becomes and the more light we have for helping others to find their innate great bright light.

The spiritual level of the practitioner directly reflects the effect of Reiki. In a sense, the more you are enlightened, the more the effectiveness of Reiki enhances.

The more you practice Reiki for saving others, the brighter your innate light shines to drive away clouds covering your mind. I think this is the quintessence of Reiki.
– Takeda Hakusai Ajari

Mikao Usui also handed us some different techniques like Byosen and Reiji-ho, tools we can utilize during a hands-on healing session. These tools also need to be seen as a meditation practice because if our mind is distracted we cannot utilize them.

Byosen is a basic technique in which we move a bit more

away from the basic standard hand positions. Reiji-ho is where we become more intuitive, letting go of labeling and ritualistic movements, allowing the energy to guide where to place your hands. These techniques help us to become more organic and true to our way and our being/True Self.

> The most basic technique in Dento Reiki [Usui Reiki Ryôhô Gakkai] involves detecting a Byosen and then placing the hands on the affected area in order to perform an effective healing treatment...Different Reiki healers experience different kinds of sensations.
> – Hiroshi Doi, *A Modern Reiki Method for Healing*

> When there are many Byosen, the technique known as Reiji-ho can be employed for greater effectiveness. Reiji-ho allows for the hands to be naturally drawn to the area that needs to be treated. This is a very important technique in Dento Reiki [Usui Reiki Ryôhô Gakkai].
> – Hiroshi Doi, *A Modern Reiki Method for Healing*

By looking at what the Usui Reiki Ryôhô Gakkai thinks of these two techniques, we can start to see that they are just stepping stones towards a full intuitive hands-on healing session without the need of any technique at all, where the energy simply guides you. This can only start to happen when we let go of our ego. Both techniques are also intuitive; when we start to label what we feel, and put that in boxes, it is counter-productive to being intuitive. These practices were placed into Mikao Usui's teachings to help us to let go of the ego, the "I." Because it is the "I" which is trying to label things as hot or cold, positive and negative, good or bad. Within true compassion there is no need to label and judge, no need to interpret what we feel. Within true compassion we can just "be." We can let the client take whatever he/she needs: not what we, the ego, thinks our client needs.

Again we reach a space of free-flowing energy and a free-flowing state of mind. The universe doesn't judge, it just flows; our True Self doesn't judge, it just flows. When we integrate all of this within our hands-on healing, then hands-on healing has become meditation.

The universal law of the great universe and one's mind must be perpetually integrated.
– Note from a student of Mikao Usui from Hiroshi Doi's manual

Chapter 28

Symbols

If we look carefully, then we realize that there are in reality only two symbols within Mikao Usui's teachings, the first two. The last two are just kanji. But why did Mikao Usui put these symbols in his teachings? They were there to be used for your own personal meditation practice. What happens when we rest our mind continuously on a symbol? We stop drifting into the past, present, and future. The symbol helps us to stay mindful of what we are doing. Normally our mind is all over the place, but by resting our mind on a symbol our mind becomes calmer and calmer. And when our mind is calm our energy becomes calm. But for this to happen we need to draw the symbol again and again and again. Drawing it once in our mind and then drifting off to the past, present, or future will not create mindfulness. Mindfulness comes when we stay focused.

Let's look at the first symbol within Okuden Level II. To draw this symbol you start at the top, horizontally, and then we go down and visualize three counterclockwise circles going inwards. If we draw this in our mind over and over then where is our mind going? Our mind is going inwards. Where is our mind normally? It is all over the place. And when our mind is all over the place our energy is also all over the place. But when we start to go inwards with our mind our energy also starts to go inwards; it starts to go home to our center, the *hara*. Thus by visualizing this symbol we become more grounded, centered and focused. So we can see that this symbol does in fact the same thing as the mantra *choku rei*, or *joshin kokyu hō*, or meditating on the precept "Do not anger." Mikao Usui created a toolbox full of techniques he could teach, depending on his student's spiritual progress and personal ways of learning.

As our mind always seems to be focused externally, our energy will naturally follow it. This means that we do not have a lot of energy within us to help us to go through difficult times in our life, we often feel depleted. However, when we bring it back home to the *hara*, internalizing it, we start to have ample energy to help us through difficult situations. This internal energy will also help us to deal with illness we encounter within our own being. It is therefore of utmost importance that we focus on the first symbol for a long period of time, until one day we "become" that symbol.

Another hidden aspect of this counterclockwise symbol is its connection to Dainichi Nyorai and Dai Kômyô. According to the esoteric teachings in Japan, the counterclockwise movement points in the direction of Dainichi Nyorai and Dai Kômyô so that one day we can embody it. Taiko Yamasaki, a Shingon priest, states in his book, *Shingon Japanese Esoteric Buddhism*, "This [counterclockwise] spiral progression represents a deepening of consciousness that eventually reaches its greatest depth with Dainichi Nyorai in the very center." Thus this symbol leads us into the direction of the center of Buddhahood, the inner heart of the precepts!

There are many layers to the symbols, but to really understand this and have the direct experience it is necessary to take an in-person class with a knowledgeable teacher who can guide you into the inner heart of these tools.

When we set anything up as the object, as something outside ourselves, right there we are conditioned by it. It does not matter how fine the object is, the result is the same. It is a deluded view, a kind of ego trip because in one way or another the ego is involved. It is very easy to be trapped there.
– Taizan Maezumi, *Appreciate Your Life: The Essence of Zen Practice*

In many modern practices the symbols are used externally, especially when we do hands-on healing on others. But does that make sense? Is this in line with the precepts, for example? Imagine a client on a table, and the practitioner performs a hands-on healing session. At the shoulder a symbol is drawn for power, and at the heart a symbol is drawn for emotional mental healing. What are we doing? We are making judgments. Is making a judgment in line with the precept of compassion?

If two practitioners treat the same person, would they draw the same symbol on the exact same spot? Probably not, because both practitioners make judgments through their own personal filters. If we make judgments, are we remembering our True Self? If we make judgments are we being open to the free-flowing universe? These are good questions to investigate for ourselves.

Limited Power

Sometimes a practitioner uses a symbol for power on a shoulder, but not on a different hand position. If we have the power within our reach, why not use it during every hand position? We might say we use our intuition to discern when to use it or not. But is our intuition always right? If we look honestly at ourselves we know that our intuition is not always right. Why limit our power if we have it? Maybe our client has an issue which we do not know of or feel, so wouldn't it be better to use this power within each hand position? However, real power is when we have become the symbol and we do not need to use something external, because real power is in the pure mind of the True Self.

Stopping judgement opens the door to wisdom.
– Maurizio Maltese, *Zen and the Art of Self Preservation: The Strategies of the Martial Arts*

Imagine a cookie jar filled with two different kinds of cookies, one cookie for power and one cookie for emotional mental healing. You go to your client and you feed your client one cookie for power and four for emotional mental healing. In your next session you feed your client two power cookies and one emotional mental cookie. You force these cookies in their mouth. Is this healthy, is this compassionate, is this kind, is this ethical? This is what we do when we draw symbols on people without their consent. Because we do not ask them, "Can I draw this here – or there?" Wouldn't it be much healthier to offer them the cookies? We could say, "Here is a jar full of cookies. Please take from it whatever you need. You want one, fine; you don't want any, that's fine too." But how do we offer? We can only offer when we let go of our own personal judgments on what our clients need. We can only offer when we have "become" the symbols. Now all we have to do is be with our client and our client can take from us whatever they need for the healing to take place.

Some might say, "But we are not forcing our symbols and energy on our clients." Think about it; we do! We draw them left, right and center, full of our judgments. Why not just learn how to become the symbols ourselves? Then we do not have to judge when to use them or not. And when our treatment is free of judgment, we are so much more open to the flow of the universe. This is why traditionally the symbols were not for healing others; they were for you, tools to remember your True Self. And when we start to slowly remember our True Self we move away from judgments and from doing Reiki, because we can now "be" Reiki.

This is also why the word Reiju, the Japanese word for initiation or attunement, translates as spiritual offering. We are offering someone the energy, the healing, and they take from this offering whatever they need. Within offering there is no need to judge, no need to draw, no need to force. Offering sets you free. Animal Reiki practitioners and teachers will clearly see what is being said here, because most animals do not like it when you force the symbols on them. They are too sensitive, too smart to let our judgments infiltrate in a treatment. They will walk or run away. However, we human beings have been numbed by putting layers of lampshades over our innate great bright light, and therefore we do not feel it when a practitioner or teacher judges when they perform a treatment.

But when we start to remember our True Self we will become aware of this, and to tell you the truth, those kinds of healings are very uncomfortable. Do we remember being judged by our teacher at school, by our parents, by our spouse, by society? How did that feel? Good and healing, or did we not like it? Remember how it feels when others judge us in our daily life, as this will help us to feel how it will be for our clients when we judge them. We might think that we do this judging because we care for our clients and that we want to help them heal themselves. But that is a very mistaken viewpoint. That viewpoint comes from the "I," the ego.

> We care about all sorts of things, and there are different kinds of caring. On a commonsense level, if your caring is right caring, then do it. If it is wrong caring, then stop it. What makes it right or wrong caring? We come back to separation, duality. If we do not see things as one, we fall into the dichotomy that creates the relative world, the right and wrong, the good and bad. Then caring is no longer true caring.
> – Taizan Maezumi, *Appreciate Your Life: The Essence of Zen Practice*

Right caring is when we have embodied Right Mind, the *hon sha ze sho nen*. Then we can really go into the heart of the system of Reiki. When we are in a state of oneness with our client there is no need to draw any symbols, just be. Some might say that we are not One yet, that we have to practice. But that statement comes from our own confused mind because in essence we have been

One with everything since conception. We just have to remember this. This is what the symbols are trying to tell us: to rediscover our True Self, which in essence is non-duality.

To sum this chapter up, traditionally the symbols were tools: signposts to point to our own True Self so that we can be free of labeling, free of judging, and One with all that is.

When we abandon the ego our consciousness opens up to the infinite.
– Taisen Deshimaru, *Mushotoku Mind: The Heart of the Heart Sutra*

Chapter 29

Signposts to Our True Self

At the beginning of this book we discussed that Reiki means True Self and within this book we have also looked at the journey from not knowing our True Self to knowing our True Self. All of Mikao Usui's methods, the precepts, symbols and mantras, the specific meditation practice, hands-on healing, and the *reiju*/initiation/ attunement are in reality signposts. These signposts are all pointing towards our True Self. However, most of the time we seem to cling to these signposts instead of looking at what they are pointing towards. In fact we are hugging the signposts and not following the path; this means we have come to a standstill, and the journey has stopped. When we cling to these signposts we forget the real reason Mikao Usui put them in his teachings. For example, we start to believe that we cannot do hands-on healing without the symbols and mantras. We start to believe that we cannot help others without hands-on healing and so on. We have become dependent on the signposts.

> All instruction is but a finger pointing to the moon; and those whose gaze is fixed upon the pointer will never see beyond. Even let him catch sight of the moon, and still he cannot see its beauty.
> – Buddha

These signposts are the famous fingers pointing towards the moon. We always discuss the signpost, yes even in this book, but by discussing it we miss the path again. Thus the real under-standing of the teachings comes from the direct experience of them, not from endlessly discussing the teachings. How do we gain this direct experience? We gain this through all the meditation practices left for us by Mikao Usui.

We also cannot always chant a mantra, do hands-on healing or sit in a specific meditation practice. How can I chant a mantra and talk to you? How can I do hands-on healing while driving my car? How can I do a specific meditation practice while running? All these practices are only there to help us to become Reiki, to remember our True Self. Remembering our True Self is a state of mind, as is indicated numerous times within Mikao Usui's teachings. And we can learn how to remember to be in that state of mind, no matter what we do. Thus the whole system of Reiki is about becoming the precepts, becoming hands-on healing, becoming the meditation practices, becoming the symbols and mantras, and becoming the *reiju*/initiation/attunement. When we have become them we can let go of all the signposts and be free, free from tools. Now we are resting our mind in the great bright light of our True Self. This is where all the signposts within the system of Reiki point.

Chapter 30

Keep Practicing

The secret of the system of Reiki is not the symbols, the mantras, or the *reiju*/initiation/attunement. The real secret is our own personal meditation practice.

This means that we need to keep meditating with the tools provided by Mikao Usui. If we do not sit down and do our practice, it will be very hard to rediscover that we are Reiki in the first place. This can only be rediscovered through a dedicated meditation practice. Some might say, "I do not need to do the meditation practices because I am channeling Reiki already," or "I have been a Reiki teacher for many years so why would I need to do these meditation practices?" We can always go deeper. The inner heart of the system of Reiki is about rediscovering our True Self, and even if we rediscover our True Self we need to keep practicing because otherwise we put the lampshades back again.

> There is always something more. If you ever sit down with a sense of "This will do", you've had it!
> – Satomi Myodo, *Passionate Journey: The Spiritual Autobiography of Satomi Myodo*

The first important elements needed within our spiritual journey are practice, patience, and perseverance. They should not be seen as separate entities, as there is an interconnectedness between them. Successful practice without patience and perseverance is not possible, and neither is perseverance without patience and the practice itself. These three need to be utilized no matter which practices we choose from the system of Reiki. Rediscovering our True Self doesn't happen overnight. It can be a long process that takes time and therefore patience is required. To keep going we need perseverance, otherwise we might stop after a while which would be a waste of our time. But to keep it all going we need to practice.

Mikao Usui used the Japanese word *gyo* within his precepts, which means practice, and he also said, "today." He gave us a hint that to really understand his teachings we need daily practice in his meditation methods. Today therefore also means every day, because every day is today.

> The value of persistence is in realizing that practice, and its benefits, can be found within everyday life. "It doesn't matter what, just find something and stick to it, that is practice (shugyo)".
> – Sakkai Yusai, in Stephen G. Covell, "Learning to Preserve: The Popular Teachings of Tendai Ascetics," *Japanese Journal of Religious Studies*, Volume 31, number 3 (2004)

The best way to create a daily meditation practice is to start slowly. A baby doesn't run straight away; she needs to discover many things before she can run. This is the same within our own personal practice. It is better to do little meditations of 5 minutes at a time, in which we are very focused, than 20 minutes in which most of the time we are thinking of the past, present, and future. Mikao Usui also said to practice daily – why? I like doing the dishes but if you leave the dishes unwashed overnight they are much harder to clean than if you wash them on the day you use them. Each day we accumulate new stuff, putting new lampshades on. If we let these sit in our system and only practice once a week it is much harder to let go of them than when we practice on the day we accumulated them. When we keep practicing we start to move from "Doing Reiki "to "Being Reiki."

> Practice (shugyo), he notes, is not simply the acquisition of knowledge, but turning that knowledge into wisdom through

experience. The foundation of "turning knowledge into wisdom" is the practice of maintaining a routine. This teaching reflects the nature of Mitsunaga's experience in the kaihogyo, and his belief in the power of persistence. Mitsunaga states that practice is all about sticking to a routine and never wavering from it. Everyday must be seen as practice. Practice is not about maintaining one's current life-style but about advancing one step at a time.

– Mitsunaga Kakudo, in Stephen G. Covell, "Learning to Preserve: The Popular Teachings of Tendai Ascetics, *Japanese Journal of Religious Studies*, Volume 31, number 3 (2004)

Chapter 31

Intimacy

As we saw in the chapter on the precepts, the kanji of kindness also means intimacy. Intimacy is a very important element, and it is also pointed out within the mantras. The quality of *sei heki* is harmony; when we are in harmony with ourselves we have become intimate with ourselves. When we are in harmony with others we have become intimate with others. When we have become in harmony with the universe we have become intimate with the universe.

> To truly understand that one and others are the same is satori.
> I and others have the same root. All beings and myself are in unity. I and the cosmos are one.
> – Taisen Deshimaru, *Mushotoku Mind: The Heart of the Heart Sutra*

This kind of intimacy is not sexual intimacy but a much deeper intimacy: it is the intimacy of our heart/mind merging with the heart/mind of all there is. You might feel this kind of intimacy when you place your hands on yourself during hands-on healing. As we discussed before, hands-on healing on yourself was added into the teachings to remember this kind of intimacy, where the toucher and the person who is touched become one. But if we keep seeing that we channel energy, or that the energy is external from ourselves, then we will not facilitate this kind of intimacy within ourselves. I know that some of you who do hands-on healing on others have felt this kind of intimacy with your client. But we can only feel this if we let go of the idea of protecting ourselves. This is why the precept "Do not worry" is utilized, because we can only reach this state of mind of intimacy when we let go of all our worries and fear. As you see, all Mikao Usui's teaching tools are interlinked with each other; they do not do separate things, they all point towards the same, our True Self. Our True Self is free of worry and always has been and will be intimate with everything there is.

> In your daily life, please accept yourself as you are and appreciate your life as it is. Be intimate with yourself. Taking good care of yourself is always the best way to take care of everything. Then your life, I am sure, will go all right. I want you to be a truly intimate being. Beneath your robe is the same as outside your robe. Inside and outside the robe are one. There is no division.
> – Taizan Maezumi, *Appreciate Your Life: The Essence of Zen Practice*

To deepen the experience of intimacy with all there is, we need to start to internalize all the methods within Mikao Usui's teachings into our heart/mind. We do this by seeing that all his tools are forms of meditation practices. Because when we meditate with the precepts, meditate with the mantras, meditate with the symbols, meditate during hands-on healing, meditate during *reiju*/initiation/attunement, then we become intimate with these tools. If we use them externally or just see them as external rituals to be performed, we will never reach intimacy. And what is real healing really about? Real healing for ourselves and others is about rediscovering this intimacy, our True Self.

Chapter 32

Doing Reiki versus Being Reiki

I often hear many people say that they are "doing Reiki," but what does that mean? Of course I know it means they are performing hands-on healing, either on themselves or on others. However, as seen throughout this book, hands-on healing is in reality only a very small part of Mikao Usui's teachings. It might be a big part in Mrs. Takata's or Hayashi's teachings, but if we practice the system of Reiki, we practice Mikao Usui's teachings! Mikao Usui's teachings are all about "Being Reiki" instead of "Doing Reiki." This is because we cannot always "Do Reiki" but we can always "Be Reiki."

Imagine you are walking down a busy shopping street. Can you walk up to each and every person, place your hands on them and *do* hands-on healing? Of course not, we would be in big trouble. But we can "Be Reiki." We can walk in that state of mind of our innate great bright light, and all the people, animals, trees, you name it, who come in contact with our innate great bright light can take from this light whatever they need. In this state, we can therefore be much more compassionate than if we keep "Doing Reiki." "Doing Reiki" is limiting, while "Being Reiki" is unlimited.

> If you want to be free, get to know your real self. It has no form, no appearance, no root, no basis, no abode, but is lively and buoyant. It responds with versatile facility, but its function cannot be located. Therefore when you look for it you become further from it, when you seek it you turn away from it all the more.
> – Zen Master Linji, in *Zen Essence: The Science of Freedom*, translated by Thomas Cleary

Did you ever have the experience of just "being" with a friend or an animal? Do you remember how it felt? No need to talk, no need for questions, no need to label and interpret things. Completely at ease, completely free. Wow, what a feeling! What if we could always be at ease. What if we could always be free. What if we could always be safe and secure. Wouldn't that be amazing? That is really what the heart of the system of Reiki is all about. This is even pointed out within the precepts, as they are not about "Doing Reiki," but rather "Being Reiki." We are not saying, "I am doing compassion" or "I am doing kindness." Rather we say, "I am being compassionate," or "I am being kind."

"Doing Reiki" is also about being busy: we always try to "do" something. And by always doing things we forget to Be. When we "Be Reiki" we are free, and we are not clinging to the signposts anymore. When we are "Doing Reiki," we also leave lots of traces. These traces are expectations that create attachments, which in turn create fear, worry, and anger. But when we "Be Reiki" we are free, no traces left. This is like a bird flying in the sky; it moves but we can't see any trace of where the bird has been. When we remember how to truly "Be Reiki" then there are no traces to be found, and we are finally completely free, like a bird, roaming the mighty sky.

Roaming the Universe
Completely Free
Be Reiki

Glossary of Japanese Terms

Anshin Ritsumei – spiritual peace in our heart/mind, enlightenment

Choku Rei – True Self, direct or straight spirit

Dai Ajari – great esoteric master

Dai Kômyô – great bright light, void, non-duality, emptiness

Darani – mantra, mystic phrase

Deshi – lineage disciple

Gakkai – society

Gassho – putting your palms together, union, non-duality

Gyo – practice, ascetic practices

Hara – stomach, center, true center, center of our True Self

Hatsurei hō – to generate a greater amount of spirit method

Hō – Dharma, method, truth, teachings

Hon sha ze sho nen – I am Right Mind, my original nature is a correct thought

Joshin – focusing the mind

Ki – energy, breath, air, life force

Kokyu – breathing, in and out breath

Ku – emptiness, void

Okuden – hidden or inner teachings

Paramitas, six – the six virtues or perfections of generosity, morality, patience, persistence, concentration, and wisdom

Reiju – spiritual blessing, spiritual offering

Reiki – True Self, spiritual energy

Ryô – to cure, to heal

Sanmitsu – three mysteries of mind, body, and speech/energy

Satori – enlightenment

Sei heki – inclination to remember our True Self

Shinpiden – mystery teachings, not just for teaching but for deepening your personal practice, remembering the mystery of the universe and life

Shoden – beginner's teachings
Tanden – field of elixir, ocean of ki
Toitsu – to unite, to unify
Waka – poetry

Bibliography

Addis, Stephen. *Zen Sourcebook: Traditional Documents from China, Korea, and Japan*, Hackett Publishing Company, Indianapolis, 2008.

Bowring, Richard. *The Religious Traditions of Japan*, Cambridge University Press, Port Melbourne, 2008.

Cleary, Thomas. *Zen Essence: The Science of Freedom*, Shambhala Dragon Edition, Boston, 2000.

Davey, H. E. *The Teachings of Tempu: Practical Meditation for Daily Life*, Michi Publishing, Albany, 2013.

Deshimaru, Taisen. *Mushotoku Mind: The Heart of the Heart Sutra*, Hohm Press, Chino-Valley, 2012.

Doi, Hiroshi. *A Modern Reiki Method for Healing*, Vision Publications, Southfield, 2014.

Gleason, William. *The Spiritual Foundations of Aikido*, Destiny Books, Rochester, 1995.

Hakeda, Yoshito S. *Kukai: Major Works*, Columbia University Press, New York, 1972.

Hyers, Conrad. *Once-Born, Twice-Born Zen: The Soto and Rinzai Schools of Japan*, Wipf & Stock Publishing, Eugene, 2004.

Katagiri, Dainin. *Each Moment Is the Universe: Zen and the Way of Being Time*, Shambhala Publications, Boston, 2007.

Katagiri, Dainin. *You Have to Say Something: Manifesting Zen Insight*, Shambhala Publications, Boston, 2000.

Kohno, Jiko. *Right View, Right Life: Insights of a Woman Buddhist Priest*, Kosei Publishing Co, Tokyo, 1998.

Kwong, Jakusho. *No Beginning, No End: The Intimate Heart of Zen*, Shambhala Publications, Boston, 2003.

Kukai. *Shingon Texts*, Numata Center for Buddhist Translation & Research, Moraga, CA, 2004.

Maezumi, Taizan. *Appreciate Your Life: The Essence of Zen Practice*, Shambhala Publications, Boston, 2002.

Maltese, Maurizio. *Zen and the Art of Self Preservation: The Strategies of the Martial Arts*, Caraba Publishing House, Milan, 2014.

Morinaga, Soko. *Novice to Master: An Ongoing Lesson in the Extent of My Own Stupidity*, Wisdom Publications, Somerville, 2002.

Myodo, Satomi. *Passionate Journey: The Spiritual Autobiography of Satomi Myodo*, Shambhala Publications, Boston, 1987.

Oda, Ryuko. *Kaji: Empowerment and Healing in Esoteric Buddhism*, Kineizan Shinjao-in Mitsumonkai, Japan, 1992.

Prasad, Kathleen. *Reiki for Dogs: Using Spiritual Energy to Heal and Vitalize Man's Best Friend*, Ulysses Press, Berkeley, CA, 2012.

Reid, Daniel. *Chi Gung: Harnessing the Power of the Universe*, Shambhala Publications, Boston, 1998.

Shaner, David Edward. *The Bodymind Experience in Japanese Buddhism*, State University of New York Press, Albany, 1985.

Shinonuma, Ryōjun. *The Life-long Spiritual Journey of an Apprentice Japanese Bonze: Awakening to a New Worldview by Fulfilling the One-thousand Days Trekking Practice on Mt. Ōmine*, Pro Sophia, Tokyo, 2014.

Smart, Ninian. *World Philosophies*, Routledge, New York, 2008.

Soho, Takuan. *The Unfettered Mind: Writings of the Zen Master to the Sword Master*, Kodansha International, Tokyo, 1986.

Stiene, Bronwen and Frans. *A–Z of Reiki Pocketbook: Everything About Reiki*, O-Books, Winchester, 2006.

Stiene, Bronwen and Frans. *The Japanese Art of Reiki*, O-Books, Winchester, 2005.

Stiene, Bronwen and Frans. *The Reiki Sourcebook*, O-Books, Winchester, 2003.

Stiene, Bronwen and Frans. *Your Reiki Treatment*, O-Book, Winchester, 2007.

Stone, Jacqueline. *Original Enlightenment and the Transformation of Medieval Japanese Buddhism*, University of Hawaii Press, Honolulu, 2003.

Suzuki, Shunryu. *Not Always So: Practicing the True Spirit of Zen*,

HarperCollins, New York, 2002.

Suzuki, Shunryu. *Zen Mind, Beginner's Mind*, Weatherhill, NY, 1970.

Unno, Taitetsu. *Shin Buddhism: Bits of Rubble Turn into Gold*, Image, 2002.

Wilson, William Scott. *The Demon's Sermon on the Martial Arts*, Kodansha International, Tokyo, 2006.

Wilson, William Scott. *The Swordsman's Handbook: Samurai Teachings on the Path of the Sword*, Shambhala Publications, Boston, 2014.

Yamakage, Motohisa. *The Essence of Shinto: Japan's Spiritual Heart*, Kodansha International, Tokyo, 2006.

Yamasaki, Taiko. *Shingon Japanese Esoteric Buddhism*, Shambhala Publications, Boston, 1988.

Yasuo, Yuasa. *The Body, Self-Cultivation, and Ki-Energy*, State University of New York Press, Albany, 1993.

Yen, Sheng. *Attaining the Way: A Guide to the Practice of Chan Buddhism*, Shambhala Publications, Boston, 2006.

Who Is Frans Stiene?

Frans has been a major influence on global research into the system of Reiki since the early 2000s. His practical understanding of the Japanese influences on the system has allowed students around the world to connect deeply with this practice.

Students naturally respond to Frans' warmth and intelligence. His own personal spiritual Reiki practice is a model that many students wish to emulate and offers great encouragement to those on the same path.

Frans is a co-founder of the International House of Reiki and Shibumi International Reiki Association with Bronwen Stiene. He has also co-authored with her the critically acclaimed books *The Reiki Sourcebook*, *The Japanese Art of Reiki*, *A–Z of Reiki Pocketbook*, *Reiki Techniques Card Deck* and *Your Reiki Treatment*.

Originally from Holland, Frans is now mainly based in Australia and since 1998 has trained in a variety of countries such as Japan, Nepal, Italy, UK and Australia. Some of his Reiki teachers include Hyakuten Inamoto, Doi Hiroshi and Chris Marsh. Frans' research has included interviewing Yamaguchi Chiyoko and other Japanese teachers, including Dr. Matsuoka. Although Frans is trained as a Gendai Reiki Ho Shihan (teacher) and a Komyo Reiki Shihan (teacher), he prefers to teach a traditional form of Japanese Reiki, Usui Reiki Ryôhô, that he feels reflects a desire to bring the teachings back to their very source, rediscovering our True Self. Most teachers in Japan teach the system of Reiki from Chujiro Hayashi's viewpoint while Frans tries to teach it as much as possible from Mikao Usui's viewpoint.

But I could find signs that he [Chujiro Hayashi] had already converted the "Usui method" into the "Hayashi method" even before he taught Takata Sensei. He seemed to try modernizing Reiki-ho based on his medical knowledge and experience as a practical therapist.

– Hiroshi Doi, *A Modern Reiki Method for Healing*

Frans is currently training with a Japanese Shingon priest, Takeda Hakusai Ajari, who was once a Tendai monk as a disciple of the great Sakai Dai Ajari, to learn about Shinto, Shugendo, Tendai, and Shingon. Frans is also studying with Reverend Yamabushi Priest Kûban from France.

Frans keeps researching and practicing traditional Japanese teachings to find out what Mikao Usui himself was practicing to get a deeper understanding about what the system of Reiki is really about. This will help him to become a better teacher and to support students in their understanding of the system and their own personal spiritual practice. Frans is one of the rare Reiki teachers who is undertaking these practices.

– Reverend Kûban Jakkôin, Shugendo priest

The contents of what Frans teaches is formed by what has been practiced in Japan since the early 1900s, long before the system of Reiki left Japan, and the researched influences on the system. This particular method includes physical and energy-enhancing exercises to help practitioners delve deeper into their Reiki practice. The earlier teachings consider the system not just to be a hands-on-healing practice but one that also focuses on a student's spiritual path.

The spiritual level of the practitioner directly reflects the effect of Reiki. In a sense, the more you are enlightened, the more the effectiveness of Reiki enhances. The more you practice Reiki for saving others, the brighter your innate light shines to drive away clouds covering your mind. I think this is the quintessence of Reiki. I hope Frans Stiene's way of understanding Reiki spreads in the world to enlighten those who practice Reiki based on a superficial understanding of the tradition.

– Reverend Takeda Hakusai

Frans' open, humorous, and informal style of teaching has been an inspiration for students and clients throughout the USA, Europe, Asia, and Australia. His aim is to provide students with the most comprehensive and up-to-date information about the system of Reiki as well as a strong energetic connection to Mikao Usui's teachings.

Apart from teaching all three levels of the system of Reiki and specialized classes, Frans offers limited one-on-one training sessions for students and one hour hands-on healing sessions all over the word. He also does one-on-one skype sessions, teaches through teleclasses, and offers retreats. During his retreats you will delve deep into rediscovering your True Self, which is a must if you want to help others. His Shinpiden Reiki III courses are attended by many existing Reiki teachers who want to take their practice to a deeper level.

For more information on all the courses, blogs etc. visit the International House of Reiki website: www.IHReiki.com

Facebook for the International House of Reiki:

www.facebook.com/IHReiki

Facebook of Frans Stiene:

https://www.facebook.com/frans.stiene

Other books co-authored by Frans Stiene and published through O-Books:

The Japanese Art of Reiki ISBN 1 905047 02 9

The Reiki Sourcebook – Revised ISBN 9781846941818

Your Reiki Treatment ISBN 1 84694 013 3

The A–Z of Reiki ISBN 1 905047 89 4

Reiki Technique Card Deck ISBN 1 905047 19 3

**AYNI
BOOKS**

"Ayni" is a Quechua word meaning "reciprocity" – sharing, giving and receiving – whatever you give out comes back to you. To be in Ayni is to be in balance, harmony and right relationship with oneself and nature, of which we are all an intrinsic part. Complementary and Alternative approaches to health and well-being essentially follow a holistic model, within which one is given support and encouragement to move towards a state of balance, true health and wholeness, ultimately leading to the awareness of one's unique place in the Universal jigsaw of life – Ayni, in fact.